IET HEALTHCARE TECHNOLOGIES SERIES 9

Human Monitoring, Smart Health and Assisted Living

Other volumes in this series:

Volume 1 **Nanobiosensors for Personalized and Onsite Biomedical Diagnosis** P. Chandra (Editor)
Volume 2 **Machine Learning for Healthcare Technologies** Prof. David A. Clifton (Editor)
Volume 3 **Portable Biosensors and Point-of-Care Systems** Prof. Spyridon E. Kintzios (Editor)
Volume 4 **Biomedical Nanomaterials: From Design to Implementation** Dr. Thomas J. Webster and Dr. Hilal Yazici (Editors)
Volume 6 **Active and Assisted Living: Technologies and Applications** Florez-Revuelta and Chaaraoui (Editors)

Human Monitoring, Smart Health and Assisted Living

Techniques and technologies

Edited by
Sauro Longhi, Andrea Monteriù and Alessandro Freddi

The Institution of Engineering and Technology

Published by The Institution of Engineering and Technology, London, United Kingdom

The Institution of Engineering and Technology is registered as a Charity in England & Wales (no. 211014) and Scotland (no. SC038698).

First published 2017

The Institution of Engineering and Technology
Michael Faraday House
Six Hills Way, Stevenage
Herts SG1 2AY, United Kingdom

www.theiet.org

British Library Cataloguing in Publication Data
A catalogue record for this product is available from the British Library

ISBN 978-1-78561-150-6 (hardback)
ISBN 978-1-78561-151-3 (PDF)

Typeset in India by MPS Limited

Contents

Editors' biographies

Sauro Longhi is a Full Professor at the Polytechnical University of Marche, Department of Information Engineering. His current teaching activities and research interests are in the area of assistive robotics, advanced smart sensors for home automation, and control systems. He has published more than 350 papers in international journals and conferences. He is the editor of three international journals in the field of robotics and control systems, coeditor of a book on Ambient Assisted Living, and scientific coordinator of several national and international research projects.

Dr. Andrea Monteriù is an Assistant Professor at the Department of Information Engineering, Polytechnical University of Marche, Italy. His research interests include theory and design of control and robotic systems, fault diagnosis and fault tolerant control, guidance and control of autonomous systems, and assistive technologies. He is involved in different research projects, he has published more than 90 papers in international journals and conferences, and he is the author of the book *Fault Detection and Isolation for Multi-Sensor Navigation Systems: Model-Based Methods and Applications* and is coeditor of two books on Ambient Assisted Living.

Dr. Alessandro Freddi is an Assistant Professor at Università degli Studi eCampus (Como, Italy), where he teaches "Instrumentation for Automation" and "System Modelling and Simulation", and is a member of the SMART Engineering Solutions & Technologies (SMARTEST) research centre. His main research activities cover fault diagnosis and fault-tolerant control with applications to robotics, and development and application of assistive technologies. He has published more than 50 papers in international journals or conferences, and is involved both in national and international research projects.

Chapter 1
Personal monitoring and health data acquisition in smart homes

Lucio Ciabattoni, Francesco Ferracuti, Alessandro Freddi, Sauro Longhi, and Andrea Monteriù

Abstract

The use of ambient assisted living technology, namely technology to improve the quality of life of people at home, is becoming a common trait of modern society. This technology, however, is difficult to be completely defined and classified, since it addresses many different human needs ranging from the physiological sphere to the psychological and social ones. In this chapter we focus on personal monitoring and data acquisition in smart homes, and propose the results of our research activities in the form of the description of three functional prototypes, each one addressing a specific need: an environmental monitoring system to measure the respiratory rate, a domotic architecture for both comfort assessment and user indoor localization, and a device for supporting mobility indoors. Each prototype description is followed by an experimental analysis and, finally, by considerations suggesting possible future developments in the very near future.

1.1 Introduction

The use of technology to improve the people's quality of life is becoming a common trait of modern society. When the technology is oriented to improve the Quality of Life (QoL) at home, it is referred to as Ambient Assisted Living (AAL). AAL technologies are typically classified according to the specific needs for which they are developed, in particular:

Physical and physiological needs This category includes the basic needs, starting from the common physiological requirements (e.g., food, drink, shelter, sleep) to prevention or treatment of illness. Technologies addressing these needs can be classified into *environmental systems* for personal monitoring, *wearable multi-sensory systems* for monitoring and measurement of physiological signals, and *intelligent robots* for continuous home care and activity monitoring.

Safety, security and comfort needs Once physiological needs are safeguarded, attention has to be paid to safety, security and comfort: everyone desires to feel at ease in his/her own living environment. Safety, security and comfort technologies can be included in the wide field of the smart home. A *smart home* can be seen as a home equipped with a system capable to manage devices, partially or totally, in order to make the home more efficient and make a more comfortable and safer life for those who live in it. The traditional smart home functions are typically divided into: *active safety*, *automatic systems*, *comfort monitoring* and *energy management*. These functions can be oriented towards assistive aims, so they are included in the assistive smart home, as a specific field of the smart home.

Autonomy needs The physical autonomy of people is of utmost importance, especially for elderly and/or impaired people. In this field, the assistive devices aim to provide: *mobility* both indoor and outdoor, *accessibility* to services and *physical rehabilitation* at home.

A complete classification would also include "Self-esteem" and "Self-actualization" needs, which are however more related to the psychological aspect and more specific to people with physical and/or mild cognitive problems, and "Social needs", which are typically addressed by using consumer hardware and software (from infotainment to communication systems [1]).

In this chapter, we provide the results of our research activities in AAL technologies for personal monitoring and data acquisition, in the form of the description of three functional prototypes belonging to each one of the three above-mentioned needs' categories. In detail, the chapter is organized as follows. Section 1.2 shows how to use an RGB-D (Red Green Blue-Depth) camera to perform the respiratory rate measurement. Section 1.3 proposes an open hardware and open software Internet of Things (IoT)-based platform, able to monitor four personal comfort parameters and provide a rough estimation of the position of a person at home. Section 1.4 presents a mobility support device, which is capable of transforming a commercial power wheelchair into an semi-autonomous navigation system. Finally, concluding remarks are reported in Section 1.5.

1.2 Respiratory rate detection using an RGB-D camera

In this section, we propose a respiratory rate measurement algorithm which makes use of an RGB-D camera [2]: this kind of device falls within the *environmental systems* for personal monitoring category, in order to satisfy physical and physiological needs, and represents one of the many possible solutions to provide human monitoring via ambient sensors. Unlike invasive methods like spirometer, pneumotachography, respiratory inductance plethysmography, thermistor or pulse oximeters [3–7], the presented method does not require a direct contact with the person to be monitored.

Several systems have been investigated in the literature: CCD camera [8], structured light plethysmography [9], slit light projection pattern [10] or ultra wide band sensors [11]. The use of RGB-D cameras for breathing detection is a quite recent technique and is described in an increasing number of articles, such as [12–22]. The algorithm proposed here automatically identifies the respiratory rate with a low-cost RGB-D camera, under different practical conditions.

1.2.1 System configuration

The proposed respiratory rate detection algorithm exploits a low-cost hardware and an open source software, and for this reason it results in a suitable solution for personal monitoring.

1.2.1.1 Hardware

An RGB-D camera is a vision sensor which can also measure the distance from a physical object (or person) within its field of view. An RGB-D camera is used for the identification of objects, even if the background and the body to recognize have the same color; moreover RGB-D cameras can recognize overlapping objects by calculating the distance to each one of them. The most adopted RGB-D cameras are based on Structured Light (SL) or Time of Flight (ToF).

SL cameras project specialized Infra Red (IR) images, which appear distorted on a 3D object. These images are captured by a normal 2D camera and analyzed, and then in-depth information is extracted. The principle of SL cameras is that, given a specific angle between emitter and sensor, the depth can be recovered from triangulation. An SL camera is composed by an IR projector, a diffraction grating and a standard Complementary Metal Oxide Semiconductor (CMOS) detector with a band-pass filter centered at the IR light wavelength. The diffraction grating is a Computer-Generated Hologram (CGH) which produces a specific periodic structure of IR light when the laser shines through it. The projected image does not change in time. The IR CMOS sensor detects this pattern projected onto the room and scene, and generates the corresponding depth image. Well-known SL cameras are the *Microsoft Kinect v1* and the *Asus Xtion*. ToF cameras rely instead on the calculation of the time which is required by an IR emission to travel from the camera to the object and back: by knowing the speed of propagation of the IR wave, it is then possible to estimate the distance. The most known ToF camera is the *Microsoft Kinect v2*.

Compared with cameras based on TOF technology, SL cameras have a shorter range, and images appear to be noisier and less accurate. Post processing algorithms can however take care of these issues. ToF cameras, instead, fail more frequently for black objects and slightly reflective surfaces. Moreover, ToF cameras are more expensive than SL cameras. More information on different camera sensors can be found in [23,24]. In the study described here we considered an SL camera, due to its affordable cost and sufficient sensor resolution, usually adequate to sense movements like those performed by the thorax during the respiratory phase [21,22,25].

1.2.1.2 Software

Open Natural Interaction (OpenNI) is used to implement further functionalities of the vision sensor. OpenNI is a multi-language and multi-platform framework that defines the Application Programming Interface (API) for writing applications that use natural interaction, i.e., interfaces that do not require remote controls but allow people to interact with a machine through gestures and words typical of human–human interactions. This API has been chosen because it incorporates algorithms for background suppression and identification of people motion, without causing a slowdown in the video.

1.2.2 Respiratory rate detection

In order to detect the respiratory rate, the person has to be identified first. This is realized by means of the *Calibration Algorithm*, already available within the OpenNI library, which recognizes different parts of the person's body, and associates a joint to each of them. After this procedure, the proposed *Respiratory Rate Detection Algorithm* starts. The *Respiratory Rate Detection Algorithm* provides the respiratory rate (breaths per minute) of the monitored person. By using the depth information provided by the camera, the algorithm identifies the person's chest and calculates the mean value of its depth at each time:

$$\bar{z}(k) = \frac{\sum_{i=1}^{N} z_i(k)}{N} \tag{1.1}$$

where $z_i(k)$ is the information about the depth of the ith point associated to the chest at sampling instant k, and N represents the number of points of the chest. The mean value $\bar{z}(k)$ is calculated by using data sampled at frequency $1/T_c$, where T_c is the sampling time. The initial position of the chest is used as the reference value, while the subsequent measurements are used to identify the number of breaths.

The algorithm calculates the weighted average of the mean values of the depth. This weighted average $\bar{z}_w(k)$ is calculated over a sliding window of m samples with the following formula:

$$\bar{z}_w(k) = \sum_{i=0}^{3} w_{(k-i)}\bar{z}(k-i) \tag{1.2}$$

where $\bar{z}$ is calculated according to (1.1) and $w_{(k-i)}$ (where $w_{(k-i)} \leq 1, \forall i \leq m$) is the weight associated to the mean value $\bar{z}(k-i)$. The choice of the sliding window size is a trade-off between noise rejection and loss of depth information caused by averaging over large window size.

After calculating the weighted average, the algorithm calculates the derivative of the weighted average as

$$d\bar{z}_w(k) = \frac{\bar{z}_w(k) - \bar{z}_w(k-1)}{T_c} \tag{1.3}$$

Equation (1.3) permits to identify the maxima and the minima of the average value, and to eliminate irregularities in breathing. The algorithm automatically analyzes the sign of the derivative, detects when it changes and checks if that sign is kept for at least n samples (robustness to disturbance). If the sign changes from negative into positive, a new breath is detected, while if the sign changes from positive into negative, the exhalation phase is detected instead.

It is also possible to extract further information from the weighted average and the derivative:

time of exhalation, $\Delta t_i^E = t_i^E - t_{(i-1)}^I$
time of inhalation, $\Delta t_i^I = t_i^I - t_{(i-1)}^E$
depth of exhalation, $\Delta \bar{z}_i^E = \bar{z}_w(t_i^E/T_c) - \bar{z}_w(t_{(i-1)}^I/T_c)$
depth of inhalation, $\Delta \bar{z}_i^I = \bar{z}_w(t_i^I/T_c) - \bar{z}_w(t_{(i-1)}^E/T_c)$

where t_i^E and t_i^I represent, respectively, the time instants at which the exhalation and the inhalation of the ith breath ends, while $\bar{z}_w(\cdot)$ is the average value of the mean values of the depth of the chest at the sampling instant in which the exhalation or the inhalation of the considered breath ends. If the person moves during the measurement, then the algorithm records the information, recalculates the position of the chest and uses it as the new reference value. Once the measurement ends, if the person moved during the acquisition, the algorithm reconstructs the mean value of the depth of the chest ($\bar{z}(\cdot)$). At the instant in which the user started to move, the mean value of the depth of the chest ($\bar{z}(\cdot)$) is shifted. In order to properly calculate the number of breaths, the algorithm sums the mean value of the signal $\bar{z}(\cdot)$ before the shift to the value of the signal $\bar{z}(\cdot)$ after the shift.

1.2.3 Experimental validation

To evaluate the performances of the proposed respiration measurement algorithm, this was tested in multiple scenarios and it proved to be robust for common domestic/home care applications [2]. A sampling frequency $1/T_c = 7$ Hz was chosen to obtain an accurate respiratory rate. The sliding window size was chosen as $m = 4$, and the weights were set to $w_k = 1$, $w_{(k-1)} = 0.7$, $w_{(k-2)} = 0.4$ and $w_{(k-3)} = 0.1$ to give more importance to the last samples. Finally the number of samples required to detect a change in the sign of (1.3) was chosen as $n = 3$.

We report here the validation test to evaluate the goodness of the algorithm w.r.t. a moving user. In order to validate our method, a spirometer was used as gold standard. During the test, participants needed to breath into a spirometer to record the respiratory course. In the meantime, the respiratory course was measured by our algorithm as well. The spirometer measures the amount of air inspired and expired through it, while the algorithm analyzes the movement of the chest. Even if the two systems measure two different breath signals (i.e., the inspired and expired air volume in the case of the spirometer, and the chest wall motion in the case of the proposed system), the measured maxima (and minima) are correlated, as it is possible to see in Figure 1.1.

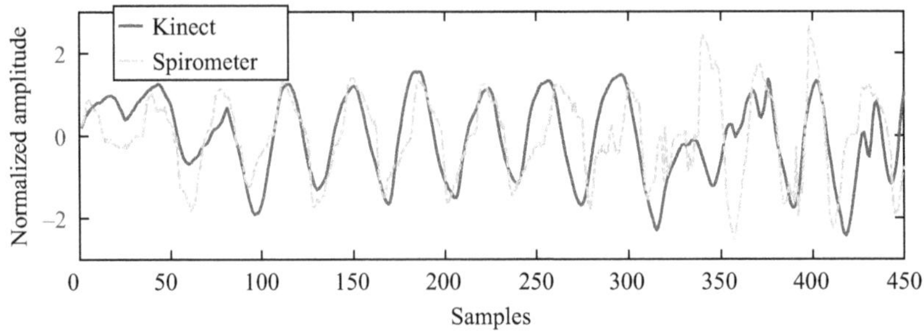

Figure 1.1 *Comparison between the normalized signals from the spirometer and from the camera. The dashed line represents the spirometer output, while the solid line that from the camera. Signals have different amplitudes, but maxima and minima match*

1.2.3.1 Setup

In these experiments, five healthy participants of both genders (three females and two males) were involved. Their age was included between 25 and 33 years old. Every participant performed three rounds of respiratory measurements. At each round, participants could breathe as they wanted (e.g., slow/fast breathing, superficial/deep breathing, etc.). We recorded the respiratory rate with our algorithm and the spirometer, and evaluated the errors coming from their comparison. Then, for each considered condition, we calculated the mean values m_i and the standard deviations σ_i of the errors for each participant $user_i$, for $i = 1, \ldots, 5$. At the end of the tests, we calculated the mean values and the standard deviations of the previous mean values for each operating condition, M and Σ, respectively:

$$M = \frac{\sum_{i=1}^{5} m_i}{5}, \quad \sum = \sqrt{\frac{\sum_{i=1}^{5} (m_i - M)^2}{5}} \tag{1.4}$$

The lower M is, the better the algorithm is. At the same time, the level of agreement between the respiratory rate measurements calculated by the proposed method and the spirometer was evaluated by using Pearson's correlation coefficient (r) and the no-correlation coefficient (p), calculated for each condition,

$$r = \frac{cov(X, Y)}{\sigma(X)\sigma(Y)}, \quad p = 2F\left(-\left|r\sqrt{\frac{n-2}{1-r^2}}\right| |n-2\right) \tag{1.5}$$

where $cov(X, Y)$ is the covariance between the two variables X and Y, $\sigma(X)$ and $\sigma(Y)$ are the standard deviations of the signals X and Y, respectively, $F(\cdot|\cdot)$ is the cumulative distribution function and n is the number of experiments. The Pearson's correlation coefficient measures the strength of linear association between two variables X and Y. The coefficient is measured on a scale with no units and can assume a value from -1 to $+1$. The higher r is and the lower p is, then the better the algorithm performs (for more details on these indexes, refer to [26,27]). The experiments were conducted

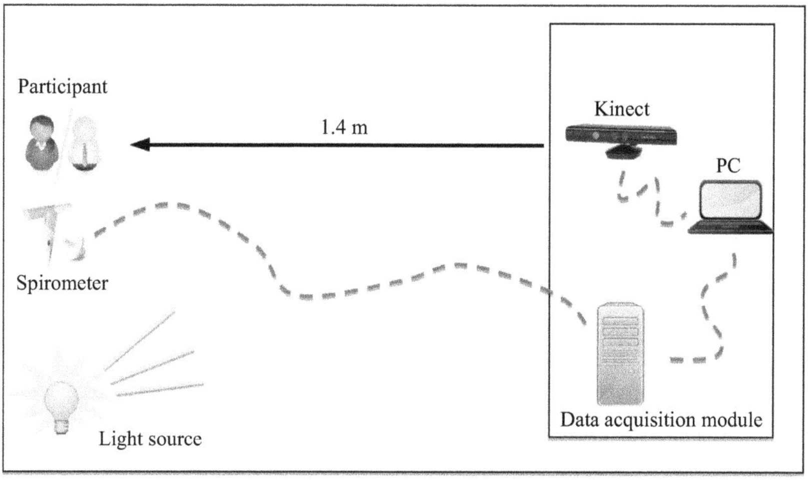

Figure 1.2 Scheme of the experimental environment in which tests were performed. The user is sitting at 1.4 m from the RGB-D camera. During the acquisition, the user has to breathe inside the spirometer and he/she can move as he/she wants on the chair

Table 1.1 Algorithm test results. m_i *= error mean value,* σ_i *= error standard deviation.* M *= mean of* m_i *values,* Σ *= standard deviation of* m_i *values.* r *= correlation coefficient,* p *= no-correlation coefficient*

Type of movement		User 1	User 2	User 3	User 4	User 5	M	Σ	r	p
Stationary	m_i	0.333	0.333	0.333	0	1	0.4	0.327	0.9802	10^{-10}
	σ_i	0.471	0.471	0.471	0	0.817				
Moving	m_i	0.333	0.333	0.667	0.333	1	0.533	0.267	0.9753	10^{-10}
	σ_i	0.471	0.471	0.471	0.471	0.817				

indoors and all participants were asked to sit at a distance of 1.4 m in front of the depth camera, as detailed in Figure 1.2.

1.2.3.2 Results

Initially, the participants were asked to remain still in front of the camera (first scenario), then they were let free to move while sitting on the chair (second scenario). Results are reported in Table 1.1.

As it is possible to see, in the worst case $M = 0.533$ and $r = 0.9753$, thus it is possible to conclude that the proposed algorithm can be used to measure the respiratory rate, both if the user is stationary or is moving. The comparison between the measurement provided by the spirometer and that provided by our systems, for a single acquisition, is reported in Figure 1.3.

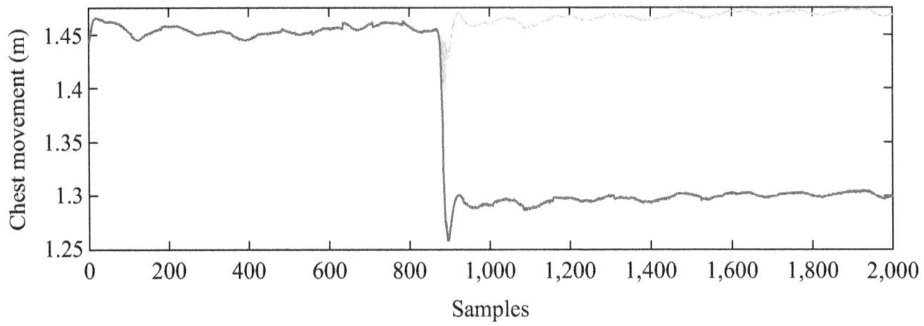

Figure 1.3 The solid line is the mean chest distance, the dashed line represents the signal after the reconstruction. As it can be seen, the algorithm reconstructs the signal to calculate the respiratory rate at the instant 880, exactly when the user moved

1.2.3.3 Considerations on the respiratory rate detection

The system has also proved to be effective against camera orientation, mild light exposure and presence of thick cloths. From a research point of view, we are currently experimenting the integration of the system with a service robot, the use of a different type of camera sensor (i.e., *Kinect v2*) and the extension of the algorithm to estimate further parameters with the aim of including it in an e-rehabilitation system for long distance therapy support.

1.3 The ComfortBox: an IoT architecture for indoor comfort monitoring and user localization

In this section, we present an Internet of Thing (IoT) architecture which can be easily integrated into a smart home, in order to provide both an assessment of the global indoor comfort and an estimation of the user position. This kind of device falls within the category of domotic systems for *comfort monitoring*, which during the last years have seen an increasing demand.

IoT opens a new realm of opportunities in the ambient monitoring scenario, due to the increasing number of connected sensors. Although comfort is a subjective concept composed by many factors (i.e., acoustical, visual, thermal and olfactory comfort) most of the recent works focus on thermal aspects only [28,29] and assess comfort condition by the use of the Predicted Mean Vote (PMV) and Percentage of Person Dissatisfied (PPD) formula [30]. Different approaches can be found in [31], where the authors proposed the monitoring of temperature, humidity and light in order to control appliances.

The solution presented in this section, namely ComfortBox [32], is an open hardware and open software IoT-based platform, which allows to monitor the four personal comfort parameters. The acoustic, olfactory, visual and thermal comfort levels are evaluated according to the international ISO, American Society of Heating,

Refrigeration and Air Conditioning Engineers (ASHRAE) and Environmental Protection Agency (EPA) regulations (standard EN15251 [33]). The platform is provided with a LightWeight Mesh 802.15.4 communication module able to manage a mesh network and interact with objects equipped with the same module. The platform is also equipped with Internet connectivity, and each object connected to the mesh network (e.g., distributed sensor or actuator) becomes remotely accessible. The integration of a personal smartwatch in the platform allows us to estimate the variables involved in the PMV formula, as well as health-related variables. In particular, we propose a method to compute a global comfort index based on a Fuzzy Inference System taking into account all the variables. Finally, we exploit the capability of each module to provide information on the Received Signal Strength Indicator (RSSI) to estimate, via software, the position of a user inside the smart home.

1.3.1 System architecture

The core system is composed by different real-world smart objects, each one equipped with an Apio General [34]. The Apio General is actually a USB stick that integrates an Atmel microcontroller with a Lightweight Mesh communication module able to create a mesh network among these objects. The gateway node is the ambient monitoring device (namely ComfortBox) and is composed by a Raspberry PI, an Apio Dongle and different sensors, i.e., a digital temperature and humidity sensor, an Indoor Air Quality (IAQ) sensor measuring carbon dioxide (CO_2) level and the concentration of Volatile Organic Compounds (VOCs), a light sensor and a microphone (temperature, humidity, indoor air quality, noise and brightness). The Apio Dongle has the same hardware specs of the Apio General but a different firmware and acts as a concentrator node. The gateway node has the task to elaborate, store and synchronize the data with the cloud.

The software platform is built using *Node.js* for both the server side and cloud synchronization while the client side is based on *Angular.js*. The non-relational database is built using *MongoDB* (the whole hardware and software structure is depicted in Figure 1.4).

Thanks to the communication module, any object equipped with a Lightweight Mesh can be connected to create a mesh network.

Since the ComfortBox is connected to the Internet (via Ethernet or Wi-Fi) any object of the mesh network can be managed via software, thus becoming remotely accessible, monitorable and/or controllable automatically through its network address and the ComfortBox IP. The smartwatch has been integrated into the system via a mobile app through a web socket: the same may apply to any smart device which is provided of wireless connection.

1.3.2 Comfort analysis

In this section we define the four different human comfort aspects, namely thermal, acoustic, visual and olfactory, as well as the related Fuzzy Sets, as shown in the following Table 1.2.

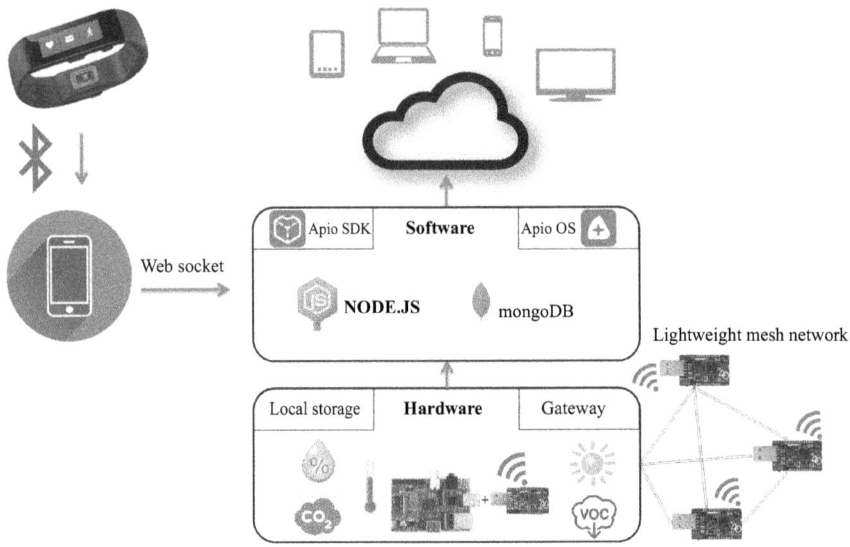

Figure 1.4 Hardware and software architecture of the ComfortBox and smartwatch communication procedure

Table 1.2 Considered fuzzy sets for the input and output variables: linguistic terms and their corresponding trapezoidal fuzzy sets

Input variables	**Linguistic terms**	**Fuzzy sets (a, b, c, d)**
Thermal Comfort (PMV)	Cold Neutral Hot	$-3, -3, -0.7, -0.5$ $-0.7, -0.5, 0.5, 0.7$ $0.5, 0.7, +3, +3$
Olfactory Comfort (ppm CO_2)	Good Bad	$0, 0, 600, 1000$ $600, 1000, +\text{inf}, +\text{inf}$
Olfactory Comfort ($\delta VOC\%$)	Low Medium High	$-100\%, -100\%, 10\%, 20\%$ $10\%, 20\%, 40\%, 50\%$ $40\%, 50\%, 200\%, 200\%$
Acoustic Comfort (dB)	Good Bad	$0, 0, 40, 60$ $40, 60, +\text{inf}, +\text{inf}$
Visual Comfort (lux)	Bad Good	$0, 0, 80, 120$ $80, 120, +\text{inf}, +\text{inf}$
Output variable	**Linguistic terms**	**Fuzzy sets (a, b, c, d)**
Global Comfort	Very low Low Medium High Very high	$0, 0, 0.1, 0.2$ $0.1, 0.2, 0.3, 0.4$ $0.3, 0.4, 0.6, 0.7$ $0.6, 0.7, 0.8, 0.9$ $0.8, 0.9, 1, 1$

1.3.2.1 Thermal comfort

The PMV/PPD model was developed by P.O. Fanger in the 1970s using heat balance equations and empirical studies about skin temperature to define comfort. Fanger's PMV equations, which can be found in [30], are based on air temperature, mean radiant temperature, relative humidity, air speed, metabolic rate and clothing insulation. Zero is the PMV ideal value and the comfort zone is defined within the recommended limits of ± 0.5 on a seven-point discrete scale from cold (-3) to hot ($+3$). According to a sensitivity analysis, the most influencing variables are the metabolic and clothing parameters, which are computed from the smartwatch measures as in [32]. We used three trapezoidal fuzzy sets to represent Thermal comfort.

1.3.2.2 Olfactory comfort

Although no standard has been set for VOCs in non-industrial settings, a warning level may be identified when VOCs value increases of a 50% with respect to its average value. At the same time it is well known [35] that CO_2 has negative effects on human working performances. It is widely reported by the technical community involved in indoor air evaluations, that the ASHRAE suggests a standard of 1,000 ppm CO_2 as the limit indoors. Concerning the olfactory aspect, two fuzzy variables have been defined.

1.3.2.3 Acoustic comfort

The noise analysis has been carried out considering the levels suggested by the Environmental Protection Agency [33] and the norm EN15251. These documents identify in 55 decibels outdoors, and 45 decibels indoors, as the levels at which oral conversation as well as other daily activities can be carried out normally.

1.3.2.4 Visual comfort

According to EPA residential illumination standards, the warning light level is around 100 lux. Two trapezoidal Fuzzy Sets have been used to model the visual comfort.

1.3.3 Fuzzy inference system

Once the different comfort aspects are assessed, we compute a global comfort index ranging from 0 (total discomfort) to 1 (optimal comfort). A five inputs – one output zero-order Takagi–Sugeno Fuzzy Inference System is used to compute the global index as shown in Figure 1.5, where 72 rules have been generated in order to obtain a single value representing the subject's comfort in the specific location. In particular, a visual feedback is generated with an RGB LED in the ComfortBox which changes its color (from blue, indicating very high comfort, to red, indicating very low comfort instead) according to the value obtained (Figure 1.6 shows a picture of the ComfortBox case).

1.3.4 RSSI-based localization

The proposed architecture is also useful for RSSI localization. RSSI is an indicator which can be used in many applications, such as the implementation of message routing or self-healing strategies for sensor networks, the detection of obstacles crossing

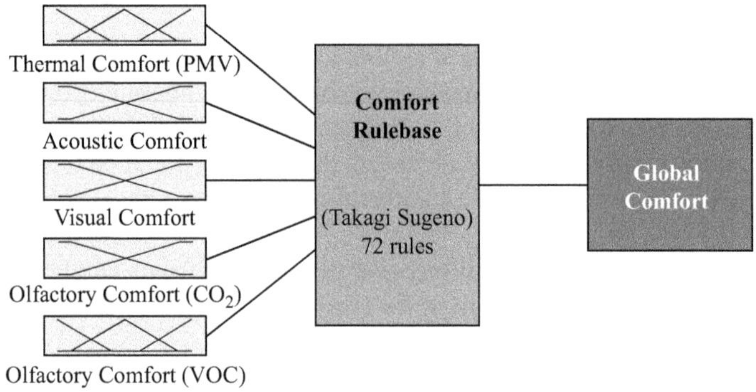

Figure 1.5 Global comfort fuzzy inference system

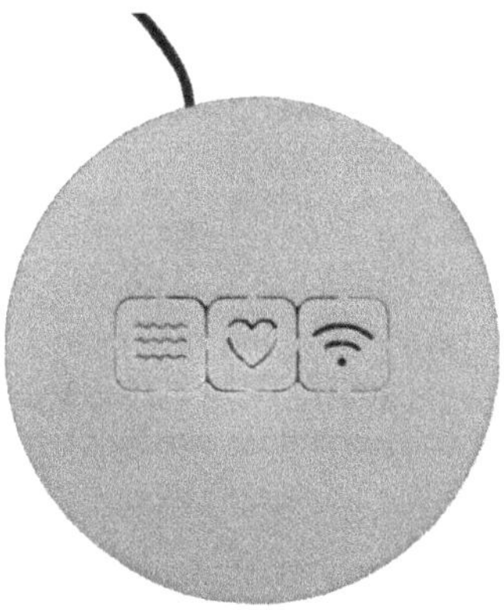

Figure 1.6 The ComfortBox case: LED lights change according to the measured global comfort

the radio-links and especially the localization of nodes. RSSI-based localization techniques rely on two different types of nodes: an Unknown Node (UN), which acts as a receiver and whose position has to be estimated, and Beacon Nodes (BNs), which act as transmitters and whose positions are known. We have developed a plug and play solution where the Apio General devices which transmit data from the smart objects are the BNs, while the UN is a generic sensor held by the user and equipped with an Apio General.

Experiments were performed by considering an area of 36 m^2 out of the total surface of the chosen test environment, composed by 16 squares with a 1.5 m side, 4 BNs in four different configurations and 1 UN. Sixteen sampled locations were identified within the environment, and their position marked on the floor. The average beacon density was 0.11 beacon nodes per square meter.

RSSI values from beacons, placed at 0.75 m from the floor, were gathered at each sampled location while the receiver was in the pocket of the user approximately at the same height of the beacons. Sixteen different tests have been performed (four for each beacon configuration).

1.3.4.1 Indoor localization algorithms

We first considered a one-slope model [36] and then used it to test three different localization algorithms, namely Min-Max, Trilateration and Maximum Likelihood. The one-slope model considers a parametric equation of the RSSI-distance (x) function, namely:

$$RSSI = A \cdot \log_{10}(x) + B \tag{1.6}$$

where RSSI is measured in power ratio dBm and x; the distance between the beacon node and the receiver node, is expressed in meters. To find the values of A and B parameters the least squares method has been considered. In particular, we performed the training of the model by considering eight tests, and the localization performances have been evaluated on the remaining eight tests: this leads to the values $A = -12.193$ and $B = -51.67$.

1.3.4.2 Experimental results

According to past researches [37], we use the Cumulative Distribution Function (CDF) of localization error to measure the localization performance. The CDF $F(e)$ of localization error e is defined in terms of a probability density function $f(e)$ as follows:

$$F(e) = \int_0^e f(x)\,dx \quad (x \geq 0) \tag{1.7}$$

From the CDF of localization error, it is possible to establish the localization error at a given confidence level (e.g., 50%, 90%). Figure 1.7 shows the cumulative probability function of the error computed for the considered scenario.

1.3.4.3 Considerations on the ComfortBox

The overall system is actually being developed to support new algorithms which should provide more accurate localization performances when the position of the BNs is known, and at least a rough information on room occupancy when that piece of information is partial or missing. The room occupancy information should then be used together with the analysis of biometric data (from the user) and the comfort data (from the ambient), in order to perform high-level correlation analysis.

1.4 A mobility support for AAL environments: the smart wheelchair

In this section, we present a device which is able to transform a classical power wheelchair into a semi-autonomous "smart" wheelchair. This kind of device falls

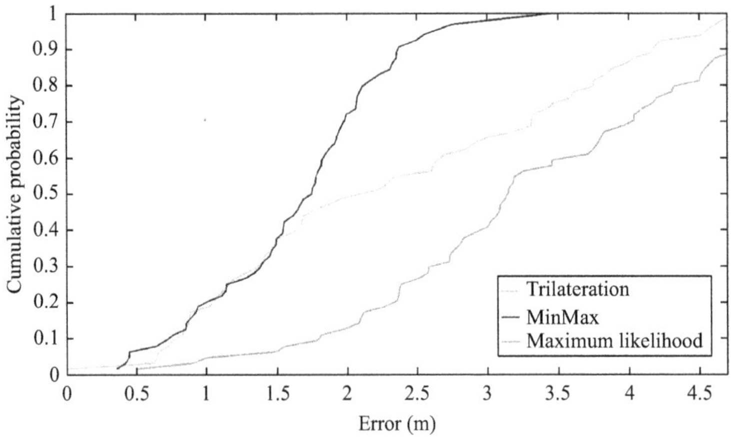

Figure 1.7 Cumulative probability computed on the validation set in the considered scenario

within the *mobility* support category, and increases the autonomy of people who are not able to walk, at least inside the home environment. Even if these devices are not strictly related to personal monitoring and health data acquisition in the present, they will be common in a near future and represent at the same time a common base both for supporting mobility and for acquiring personal data for many impaired and/or elderly people [38].

The smart-wheelchair field is one of the main research topics in AAL area [39,40]. In the last 30 years several solutions were proposed and developed in order to realize a more easy and useful system to equip standard commercial wheelchair [41]. The main features shared between these different solutions are related to the kind of sensors and the algorithms exploited. Usually, the developed localization system for AAL applications are characterized by the presence of proprioceptive (inertial measurement unit, encoder), exteroceptive (laser scanner, sonar) sensors [42] and an elaboration unit [43]. These sensors allow us to realize the typical set of navigation tasks, like localization, path planning and following, obstacle avoidance. These tasks are possible thanks to the implementation of navigation algorithms (odometric localization, Monte Carlo localization) running on an elaboration unit, typically a personal computer [44].

The developed navigation system, i.e., system which permits the wheelchair to automatically move from one place to another, is realized through a compact embedded platform, that replaces the personal computer elaboration unit. The selected embedded board permits to realize the needed computation effort in a small hardware, without introducing a cumbersome elaboration unit on the little space available on the vehicle. This innovation would permit us to realize an economic localization system, preserving every needed functionality, and easy customizable for a great number of power wheelchair producers.

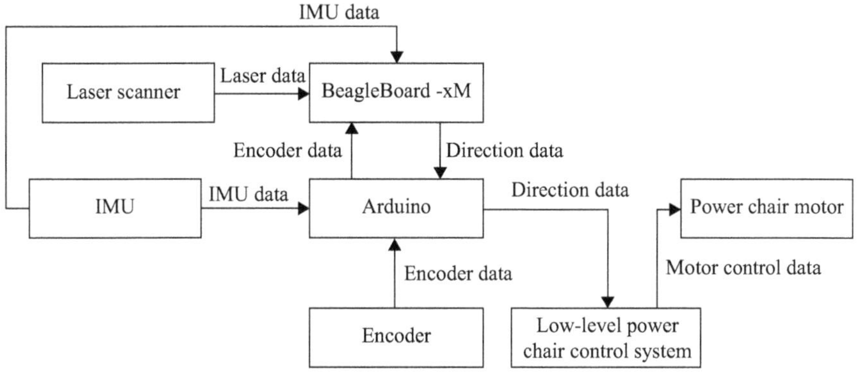

Figure 1.8 Hardware setup of the wheelchair navigation system

1.4.1 System setup

The prosed solution is realized by a commercial power chair (Sunrise Medical Quickie Salsa R2) equipped with the following sensors:

- Inertial measurement unit (IMU) Microstrain 3DMGX2-25;
- laser scanner Hokuyo UTM-30LX;
- encoders Sicod F3-1200-824-BZ-K-CV-01.

In addition two low-cost embedded platforms are used:

- Arduino Mega micro-controller;
- BeagleBoard -xM embedded board.

The BeagleBoard [45] is equipped with Ubuntu 14.04 LTS operating system, and the navigation system is developed working with the Robotic Operating System (ROS) framework [46]. The Arduino board [47] is used like a gateway that accounts for the communication between BeagleBoard -xM board, sensors (encoders) and actuators (internal power chair motor control system). The complete hardware system scheme is shown in Figure 1.8. The encoders and the IMU allow to solve the inertial localization (dead reckoning problem) problem by combining their data by an odometric algorithm based on the Kalman filter (KF). The rest of the developed navigation system is the ROS navigation stack, supplied by ROS community, based on the Adaptive Monte Carlo Localization (AMCL) algorithm. This is an open source package, customized by the authors for this kind of AAL scenario application. The software system is then based on the ROS framework paradigm, with the division of the elaboration between nodes and the nodes communication realized by topics (Figure 1.9). Each node represents a single algorithm, implemented as stand-alone and running like an autonomous tread. Each topic realizes a communication channel for data elaborated and shared between nodes, and can contain only an exact data type, and could be written and read by any node in the system.

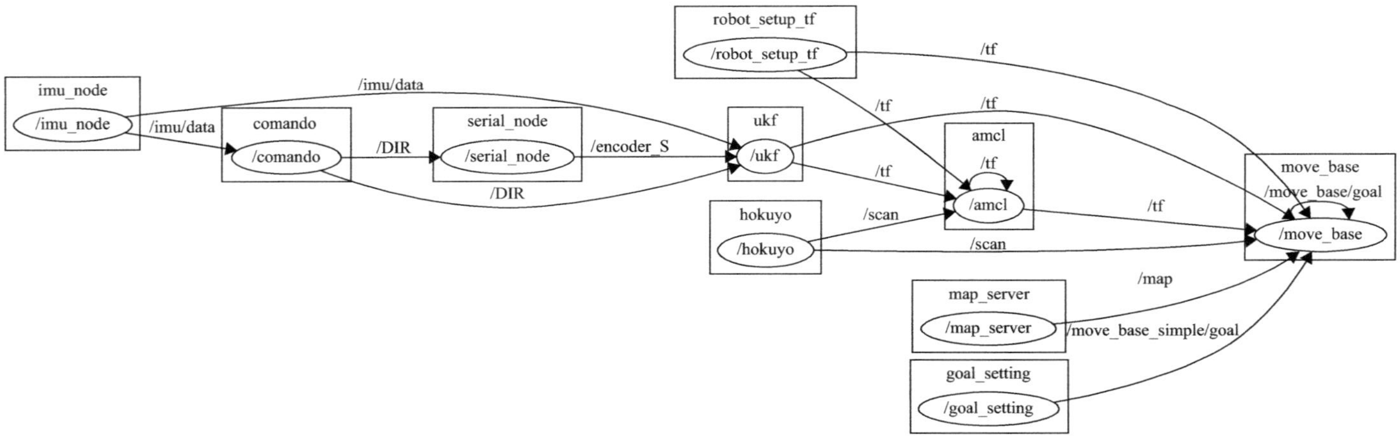

Figure 1.9 Software setup of the wheelchair navigation system

Table 1.3 Closed loop test error

Algorithm	Average closed-loop error [m]
EKF	0.0762
UKF	0.0864

1.4.2 Experimental results

The results proposed in this subsection are related to the localization, path following and obstacle avoidance algorithms.

1.4.2.1 Localization

The proposed results show the difference in terms of medium localization errors obtained using two algorithms during a closed loop test, on a distance of 16 m repeated 5 times. The odometric estimation is realized with a rate of 20 Hz, that is the encoder data acquisition frequency. Local map reconstruction occurs at a frequency of 5 Hz. Global map localization data is computed combining odometric estimation and local map data. It is updated at a 2 Hz rate. The algorithms tested in this section are based on the Extended Kalman Filter (EKF) and the Unscented Kalman Filter (UKF) characterized by 5 sigma points. In both algorithms, the orientation IMU data are considered as parameters, since the orientation data are characterized by a covariance very small respect to the covariance of the encoders data [44]. The numerical results are reported in Table 1.3.

1.4.2.2 Path following and obstacle avoidance

A set of tests was realized to validate the system during the obstacle avoidance, path planning and path following task as well. In particular, the vehicle, placed in an unknown position, starts the localization task and finds its correct position (usually within 5 s). Then the path planning and following is tested by sending to the wheelchair a valid goal into the static map. The wheelchair elaborates a valid path, and during the run, it manages the presence of obstacles, recalculating the path up to reach the desired final position. The tested obstacles are static objects unknown into the static map, and dynamic obstacles represented by people walking in front of the vehicle (which is the common case in assistive scenarios). In the first case, the wheelchair avoids the static obstacle with a modified path; in the second case, it stops at the distance imposed during the algorithm set-up. In both cases, after the correct obstacle avoidance, the wheelchair reaches the correct final position.

1.4.2.3 Considerations on the smart wheelchair

The research on the smart wheelchair is actually focusing on the integration of aid measurements which could prove useful indoors. In particular, we are integrating computer vision for artificial landmark recognition (e.g., QR codes) in order to reset the odometry error with time and improve the localization performances. From an assistive point of view, we are actually improving the user interface, in order to allow the wheelchair user to select the set-point to which navigate directly from an interactive map available on a smart device (e.g., a tablet). Moreover, we are integrating a complementary set of sensors able to acquire personal data of the user, such that to improve his/her safety and his/her usability experience of the wheelchair.

1.5 Conclusions

In this chapter we have shown the results of our research in AAL technologies for personal monitoring and data acquisition, in the form of the description of three functional prototypes developed within the laboratories of the Information Engineerig Department at Università Politecnica delle Marche in Ancona (Italy).

First, we have proposed a system, based on an RGB-D camera, to measure the respiratory rate: it belongs to the *environmental systems* for personal monitoring category, and represents one possible way of dealing with *physical and physiological needs* by using assistive technology. Then, we have proposed an IoT architecture for the comfort assessment and user indoor localization: this falls within the category of domotic systems for *comfort monitoring*, and gives an idea of how state-of-the-art home (and building) automation systems can satisfy safety, security and comfort needs. Finally, we presented a device for supporting mobility indoors, in detail a navigation system for power wheelchairs: this kind of device falls within the *mobility* support category with the aim to satisfy the need of autonomy of people with mobility problems. In this last case, the problem may not seem directly connected to personal monitoring and data acquisition; however, if we take into account elderly people, the situation becomes clearer. Elderly live often alone today and even if they conduct an independent daily life, some of them move with the aid of walkers or using wheelchairs. Monitoring elderly activity in mobility has become a major priority to provide them an effective care service, and smart wheelchairs will probably be the main platform for data acquisition of people with mobility problems in a next future.

At the end of each section we also provided some considerations on each of the presented systems, with the aim of giving an idea of possible future developments in the very next future.

Acknowledgments

We would like to thank Dr. F. Benetazzo, G. Cimini and L. Cavanini for their support in the design of the prototypes described in this chapter.

References

[1] F. Benetazzo, F. Ferracuti, A. Freddi, *et al.*, "AAL technologies for independent life of elderly people," in *ser. Biosystems & Biorobotics, Ambient Assisted Living: Italian Forum 2014*. Switzerland: Springer International Publishing,

Jul. 2015, vol. 11, pp. 329–343, e-ISBN: 978-3-319-18374-9, ISBN: 978-3-319-18373-2, ISSN: 2195–3562.

[2] F. Benetazzo, A. Freddi, A. Monteriù, and S. Longhi, "Respiratory rate detection algorithm based on RGB-D camera: theoretical background and experimental results," *IET Healthcare Technology Letters*, vol. 1, no. 3, pp. 81–86, Sep. 2014, e-ISSN: 2053–3713.

[3] K. F. Whyte, M. Gugger, G. A. Gould, J. Molloy, P. K. Wraith, and N. J. Douglas, "Accuracy of respiratory inductive plethysmograph in measuring tidal volume during sleep," *Journal of Applied Physiology*, vol. 71, no. 5, pp. 1866–1871, 1991.

[4] J. P. Cantineau, P. Escourrou, R. Sartene, C. Gaultier, and M. Goldman, "Accuracy of respiratory inductive plethysmography during wakefulness and sleep in patients with obstructive sleep apnea," *Chest*, vol. 102, no. 4, pp. 1145–1151, 1992.

[5] A. BaHammam, "Comparison of nasal prong pressure and thermistor measurements for detecting respiratory events during sleep," *Respiration*, vol. 71, no. 4, pp. 385–390, 2004.

[6] N. Douglas, S. Thomas, and M. Jan, "Clinical value of polysomnography," *The Lancet*, vol. 339, no. 8789, pp. 347–350, 1992.

[7] P. Leonard, T. Beattie, P. Addison, and J. Watson, "Standard pulse oximeters can be used to monitor respiratory rate," *Emergency Medicine Journal*, vol. 20, no. 6, pp. 524–525, 2003.

[8] K. Nakajima, Y. Matsumoto, and T. Tamura, "Development of real-time image sequence analysis for evaluating posture change and respiratory rate of a subject in bed," *Physiological Measurement*, vol. 22, no. 3, pp. N21–N28, 2001.

[9] R. Wareham, J. Lasenby, P. Cameron, and R. Iles, "Structured light plethysmography (SLP) compared to spirometry: a pilot study," in *European Respiratory Society Annual Congress*, Vienna, Austria, 2009.

[10] H. Aoki and K. Koshiji, *Non-contact Respiration Monitoring Method for Screening Sleep Respiratory Disturbance Using Slit Light Pattern Projection*. Berlin, Heidelberg: Springer, 2007, pp. 680–683.

[11] E. M. Staderini, "UWB radars in medicine," *IEEE Aerospace and Electronic Systems Magazine*, vol. 17, no. 1, pp. 13–18, Jan. 2002.

[12] N. Burba, M. Bolas, D. M. Krum, and E. A. Suma, "Unobtrusive measurement of subtle nonverbal behaviors with the Microsoft Kinect," in *IEEE Virtual Reality Workshops*, Costa Mesa, California, March 2012, pp. 1–4.

[13] M. Martinez and R. Stiefelhagen, "Breath rate monitoring during sleep using near-IR imagery and PCA," in *21st International Conference on Pattern Recognition*, Tsukuba Science City, Japan, Nov. 2012, pp. 3472–3475.

[14] M. C. Yu, J. L. Liou, S. W. Kuo, M. S. Lee, and Y. P. Hung, "Noncontact respiratory measurement of volume change using depth camera," in *2012 Annual International Conference of the IEEE Engineering in Medicine and Biology Society*, San Diego, California, Aug. 2012, pp. 2371–2374.

[15] M.-C. Yu, H. Wu, J.-L. Liou, M.-S. Lee, and Y.-P. Hung, "Breath and position monitoring during sleeping with a depth camera," in *Proceedings of*

the International Conference on Health Informatics, Vilamoura, Algarve, Portugal, 2012, pp. 12–22.
[16] J. Xia and R. Siochi, "A real-time respiratory motion monitoring system using Kinect: proof of concept," *Medical Physics*, vol. 39, no. 5, pp. 2682–2685, 2012.
[17] E. A. Bernal, L. K. Mestha, and E. Shilla, "Non contact monitoring of respiratory function via depth sensing," in *IEEE International Conference on Biomedical and Health Informatics*, Valencia, Spain, June 2014, pp. 101–104.
[18] M.-Z. Poh, D. McDuff, and R. Picard, "Non-contact, automated cardiac pulse measurements using video imaging and blind source separation," *Optics Express*, vol. 18, no. 10, pp. 10762–10774, 2010.
[19] S. Kumagai, R. Uemura, T. Ishibashi, *et al.*, "Markerless respiratory motion tracking using single depth camera," *Open Journal of Medical Imaging*, vol. 6, no. 1, p. 20, 2016.
[20] W.-C. Liao, H.-H. Lin, H.-L. Ruo, and P.-H. Hsu, "A multimedia system for breath regulation and relaxation," *International Journal of Advanced Computer Science and Applications*, vol. 6, no. 12, pp. 56–63, 2015.
[21] Q. V. Tran, S.-F. Su, and M.-C. Chen, "Breath detection for enhancing quality of x-ray image," in *International Conference on System Science and Engineering*. Nan Tou County, Taiwan: IEEE, 2016, pp. 1–4.
[22] J. Wheat, S. Choppin, and A. Goyal, "Development and assessment of a Microsoft Kinect based system for imaging the breast in three dimensions," *Medical engineering & physics*, vol. 36, no. 6, pp. 732–738, 2014.
[23] B. Mrazovac, M. Z. Bjelica, I. Papp, and N. Teslic, "Smart audio/video playback control based on presence detection and user localization in home environment," in *Second Eastern European Regional Conference on the Engineering of Computer Based Systems*, Bratislava, Slovakia, Sep. 2011, pp. 44–53.
[24] S. Song, S. P. Lichtenberg, and J. Xiao, "SUN RGB-D: a RGB-D scene understanding benchmark suite," in *The IEEE Conference on Computer Vision and Pattern Recognition*, Boston, MA, USA, Jun. 2015.
[25] K. Khoshelham and S. O. Elberink, "Accuracy and resolution of Kinect depth data for indoor mapping applications," *Sensors*, vol. 12, no. 2, p. 1437, 2012.
[26] J. Benesty, J. Chen, Y. Huang, and I. Cohen, *Pearson Correlation Coefficient*. Berlin, Heidelberg: Springer, 2009, pp. 1–4.
[27] L. Hatcher and S. Institute, *Step-by-step Basic Statistics Using SAS®: Exercises*, ser. Step-by-step Basic Statistics Using SAS®. SAS Institute, 2003.
[28] A. Pourshaghaghy and M. Omidvari, "Examination of thermal comfort in a hospital using PMV-PPD model," *Applied Ergonomics*, vol. 43, no. 6, pp. 1089–1095, 2012.
[29] L. Ciabattoni, G. Cimini, F. Ferracuti, M. Grisostomi, G. Ippoliti, and M. Pirro, "Indoor thermal comfort control through fuzzy logic PMV optimization," in *International Joint Conference on Neural Networks*, Killarney, Ireland, Jul. 2015.

[30] ISO (International Standard Organization), "ISO-7730:2006 norm," (https://moodle.metropolia.fi/pluginfile.php/217631/mod_resource/content/1/EVS_EN_ISO_7730%3B2006_en.pdf), 2007, last access December 18, 2014.

[31] S. Kelly, N. Suryadevara, and S. Mukhopadhyay, "Towards the implementation of IoT for environmental condition monitoring in homes," *Sensors Journal, IEEE*, vol. 13, no. 10, pp. 3846–3853, Oct. 2013.

[32] L. Ciabattoni, F. Ferracuti, G. Ippoliti, S. Longhi, and G. Turri, "IoT based indoor personal comfort levels monitoring," in *IEEE International Conference on Consumer Electronics*, Berlin, Germany, 2016, pp. 125–126.

[33] E. P. Agency, "Information on levels of environmental noise requisite to protect public health and welfare with an adequate margin of safety," (https://www.rosemonteis.us/files/references/usepa-1974.pdf), 1974, last access January 25, 2017.

[34] APIO, "APIO SRL official website," (http://www.apio.cc), 2015, last access January 25, 2017.

[35] U. Satish, M. J. Mendell, and K. Shekhar, "Is CO_2 an indoor pollutant? Direct effects of low-to-moderate CO_2 concentrations on human decision-making performance," *Environmental Health Perspectives*, vol. 120, no. 12, pp. 1671–1677, 2012.

[36] M. A. Panjwani, A. L. Abbott, and T. S. Rappaport, "Interactive computation of coverage regions for wireless communication in multifloored indoor environments," *IEEE Journal on Selected Areas in Communications*, vol. 14, no. 3, pp. 420–430, 1996.

[37] X. Luo, W. J. OBrien, and C. L. Julien, "Comparative evaluation of received signal-strength index (RSSI) based indoor localization techniques for construction jobsites," *Advanced Engineering Informatics*, vol. 25, no. 2, pp. 355–363, 2011, information mining and retrieval in design.

[38] C. Ma, W. Li, R. Gravina, and G. Fortino, "Activity recognition and monitoring for smart wheelchair users," in *20th International Conference on Computer Supported Cooperative Work in Design*. Nanchang, China: IEEE, 2016, pp. 664–669.

[39] M. Hillman, "2 rehabilitation robotics from past to present – a historical perspective," in *Advances in Rehabilitation Robotics*. Berlin: Springer, 2004, pp. 25–44.

[40] A. Lankenau and T. Röfer, "Smart wheelchairs – state of the art in an emerging market," *Zeitschrift Kunstliche Intelligenz*, vol. 14, no. 4, pp. 37–39, 2000.

[41] R. C. Simpson, "Smart wheelchairs: a literature review," *Journal of Rehabilitation Research and Development*, vol. 42, no. 4, p. 423, 2005.

[42] J. Borenstein, H. R. Everett, L. Feng, and D. Wehe, "Mobile robot positioning-sensors and techniques," DTIC Document, Tech. Rep., 1997.

[43] R. Simpson, E. LoPresti, S. Hayashi, I. Nourbakhsh, and D. Miller, "The smart wheelchair component system," *Journal of Rehabilitation Research and Development*, vol. 41, no. 3B, p. 429, 2004.

[44] L. Cavanini, F. Benetazzo, A. Freddi, S. Longhi, and A. Monteriù, "SLAM-based autonomous wheelchair navigation system for AAL scenarios," in

Proceedings of the IEEE/ASME 10th International Conference on Mechatronic and Embedded Systems and Applications (MESA), Senigallia, Italy, Sep. 2014, ISBN: 978-1-4799-2772-2.

[45] Beagleboard, "Beagleboard official website," (http://www.beagleboard.org/), 2016, last access January 25, 2017.

[46] ROS, "Robot Operative System official website," (http://www.ros.org/), 2016, last access January 25, 2017.

[47] Arduino, "Arduino official website," (http://www.arduino.cc), 2016, last access January 25, 2017.

Chapter 2

Contactless monitoring of respiratory activity using electromagnetic waves for ambient assisted living framework: feasibility study and prototype realization

Valerio Petrini, Valentina Di Mattia, Alfredo De Leo, Lorenzo Scalise, Paola Russo, Giovanni Manfredi, and Graziano Cerri

Abstract

Respiratory rate is a vital parameter of primary importance in medicine, sport/fitness and wellness in general, especially for most vulnerable categories of people like children and elderly people. Contactless determination of breathing activity provides a powerful and essential mean for evaluating this parameter in subjects who cannot accommodate physical sensors on their bodies. In hospital such subjects may be intensive care patients, prematurely born children and hosts of burn units. Moreover, also for long-term measurements of healthy people, for example, an elder living in home alone or in a care centre, invasive systems prove to be uncomfortable and annoying. Even for a night-time diagnosis of respiratory sleep disorders, like apnoea and hypopnoea, they demonstrate to interfere with the sleep regularity. Therefore, in the last decades many electronic devices have been conceived and realized to detect such an important parameter along with different branches of physics: strain gauges, ultrasounds, optics, thermometry, etc. This chapter presents the theoretical studies, the design and realization of a standalone Electromagnetic (EM) system for contactless determination of breathing frequency and subject's activity. Two major EM solutions are already known in the literature, continuous wave (CW) systems, and ultra-wideband (UWB) systems. The first evaluates the Doppler effect caused by the chest displacement during breathing at a single frequency, and the other one is a radar that detects the body motion by measuring the time shifts of sequential pulses. An intermediate solution that joins the advantages of both and overcomes their drawbacks is proposed. Through the use of a frequency sweep, in fact, it is possible to retrieve the equivalent information that UWB pulses are able to give, yet keeping the same contained hardware complexity of a CW system. At the same time, the proposed system proves to be robust and insensible to environmental changes. The theoretical studies have aimed at the demonstration that the solution under study helps in avoiding the blind frequencies that affect CW systems, because of sensitivity issues that depend on the variability of the reflection coefficient from the frequency and, as proved, from the harmonic content of the monitored motion. Supported by such theoretical studies, the preliminary tests are performed using laboratory instrumentation (a VNA and a commercial double ridge antenna) for a thorough campaign of measurements on assorted frequency bands, both in a controlled environment (anechoic angle) and in a concrete house, that inherently clutter the received signal. The second step involves the design and realization of a custom antenna, to be used in place of the double ridge and operating in a narrower band, which has demonstrated the same reliability of the commercial one. It has been verified in different conditions that the proposed system is able to detect both the position of the subject (i.e. distance from the antenna) and his breathing frequency, without any need for collaboration from the subject under measure. The final activity is the realization of a prototype of the device that implements the algorithms that have been studied. It is worth to highlight that the proposed system can be profitably adopted for Ambient Assisted Living framework, since it is not invasive and does not infringe the privacy of the end user, and yet it provides many valuable information about the subject's health status.

2.1 Introduction: state of the art on breathing monitoring

Respiratory activity is one of the fundamental vital signs of a human being. The respiration acts, their frequency and eventual suspension or sudden rate variations are parameters typically monitored in hospitalized patients, particularly in intensive care units, together with the heart rate, arterial pressure, etc. In a medical environment, important applications are the monitoring of respiratory-related pathologies, as the obstructive sleep apnoea syndrome (OSAS), which affect 4% of adult males, and the sudden infant death syndrome (SIDS), which represents the third leading cause of infant mortality.

Nowadays, monitoring of breathing activity is becoming a process of primary interest not only for patients in hospitals, but also for subjects living at home and requiring a remote control of their physiological status [1]. For a domestic application, the classical hospital monitoring instrumentation, like spirometer or a surveillance video system, has the disadvantage of being invasive and not respectful of the privacy of the patient. On the other hand, the use of an electromagnetic (EM)-based solution [2] has the advantage of being contactless and suitable for dressed people, since EM waves can penetrate clothes, yet ensuring the privacy of the end user.

There are many devices that can be used for monitoring the breathing activity of a subject. They can be divided into two categories: those which make use of typical EM quantities (waves and impedance changes), and those which do not. Another distinction could be made according to the invasiveness of the sensor: devices that require some kind of contact with the subject under measure (i.e. to wear belts, electrodes, to be confined on a bed or armchair) and devices whose use can be

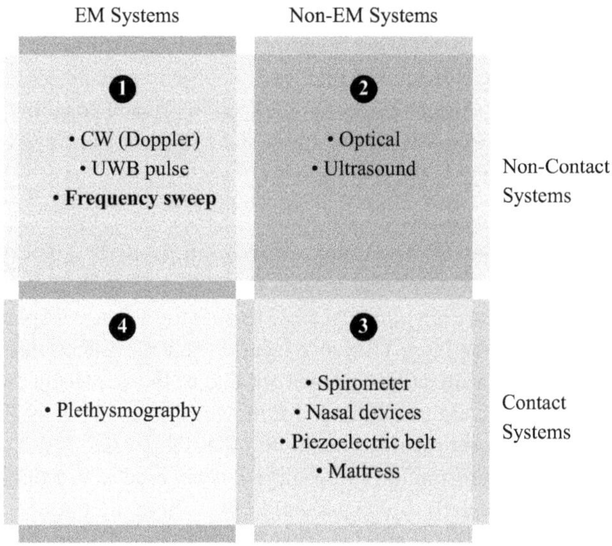

Figure 2.1 Classification of breathing detection methods

transparent for the subject. Therefore as depicted in Figure 2.1 we could define four categories of sensors, briefly described in the next subsections.

2.1.1 Non-EM and/or contact systems

This section outlines those systems that belong to categories ***2***, ***3*** and ***4*** of Figure 2.1, while the category ***1*** will be detailed in the next section.

Category **2***: Optical sensors*

The effectiveness of optical measurement for both breathing and heart rate detections has been demonstrated in [3], where a study on 55 baby patients recovered in a Neonatal Intensive Care Unit has been carried out using a Laser Doppler Vibrometer (LDVi). Comparison with a spirometer and ECG data has also pointed out that differences are below 3% for breathing rate and <6% as concern ECG data. The same principle is used in [4], where the interferometric laser setup is used to detect vibration of the skin surface caused by heart pulses on the carotid area, radial, and dorsal pedal arteries.

One drawback of a laser system is that it is punctual, therefore strongly dependent on the position of the subject with respect to the beam.

Furthermore, such a system needs direct access to subject's skin: if the subject wears loose clothes the heart beat is completely lost and also the detected chest excursion is strongly influenced.

A thermometric approach using an IR single-point temperature sensor is shown in [5], where the beam area is wider but must be pointed to the face of the subject to detect temperature variations caused by air flow during breathing.

By using fibre grating 3D sensors as described in [6], it is possible to estimate the volume change of the chest during breathing. This system projects a grid of bright points on the body of the subject and then two video-cameras detect the motions of such points. Of course the use of cameras may lead to privacy concerns and their use is intended only for intensive care units where the subject is confined on a bed with his/her chest directed towards the two cameras.

Category **2**: *Ultrasonic sensors*
Another kind of contactless systems makes use of ultrasounds (US). The studies of Min *et al.* [7,8] describe systems that rely on the US wave reflection over the body. Therefore, these systems are not punctual and measure the average displacement of the chest/belly area during breathing. They also clearly show the difficulties in measuring the respiration when the subject has clothes on, due to the scattering and absorption of sound wave by the texture of clothing. Moreover, it is shown that different kinds of texture provides different results, concluding that the system is not able to detect sufficient body motion information if the subject is covered with a thick blanket. An original application (patented) is also present in [9], where the frequency shift of the US wave is used to detect the emitted air flow coming from the mouth or the nose of the subject. In this case, the velocity difference between the air inhaled (or exhaled) and the ambient environment produces the Doppler effect.

Category **3**: *Spirometer*
The spirometer is the only system that provides a direct measurement of respiration, since it effectively detects the net air exchanged volume during breathing. Lung diseases like asthma, bronchitis and emphysema can be discriminated from tests using a spirometer. A measurement session made with the spirometer requires the subject to put a clip on his nose and breath into a mouthpiece. Then, it is an essential diagnostic instrument but its invasiveness does not allow its use for long-term measurements.

Category **3**: *Nasal devices*
These systems usually rely on a nasal cannula that measures the air flowing from the nose [10] or on a thermocouple/thermistor that detects the temperature variation caused by the emission of air [11] in the anterior naris area. This latter approach is demonstrated to be a little less sensible than air flow measurement [12].

Category **3**: *Piezoelectric belt*
A respiratory belt transducer contains a piezoelectric device that responds linearly to changes in length. It measures variations of thoracic or abdominal circumference during respiration and is able to indicate inhalation, expiration, and breathing strength [13]. However, it may be uncomfortable, and may interfere with a regular sleep. It is also not suitable for severely burned people or prematurely born children.

Category **3**: *Mattress*
These systems work only when the subject is in bed. It is basically an additional mattress that is placed under the subject or under the conventional one. It can be [14]:

- air mattress [15,16]
- capacitive sensor [17]

- piezoelectric sensor [18]
- load cell sensor sheet [19] or placed on the bed supports [20]
- static charge sensor [21,22]
- fibre-optic pressure sensor array [23]

In every case a variation of pressure, capacity, or voltage is used to estimate the movements associated with breathing. The definition of signal-to-noise ratio used in [15] has been adopted (with minor differences) during the EM signal processing described in this chapter.

Category **4**: *Plethysmography*
The interface of Respiratory Inductance Plethysmography (RIP) may be considered similar to the one of the belt, except that instead of measuring a mechanical variation of belt length, a variation of impedance is detected. It may be composed of a single belt or two belts [24]. In the latter case two sinusoidal shaped insulated wire coils are positioned within two 2.5 cm wide, lightweight elastic bands. The transducer bands are positioned around the rib cage under the armpits and around the abdomen at the level of the belly. They are connected to an oscillator and subsequent frequency demodulation electronics to obtain digital waveforms. During inspiration the cross-sectional area of the rib cage and abdomen increases altering the self-inductance of the coils and the frequency of their oscillation. The electronics convert this change in frequency to a digital respiration waveform whose amplitude is proportional to the inspired breath volume.

Another solution exploiting a similar principle involves a coil placed under the bed, fed by an LR oscillator [25]. The conductivity changes of the lungs during breathing produces a variation in the impedance seen by the oscillator loop that slightly modifies its frequency. Of course this method is extremely sensible to patient's movements and also strongly dependent on the distance and position of the body from the sensor. Furthermore it has been tested under deep breathing conditions, then according to the authors themselves, its sensitivity could be improved.

The evaluation of Transthoracic Electrical Impedance allows a plethysmography measurement using electrodes instead of belts. In [26] are described the results for an instrument with four electrodes, one placed at the top of the neck and another at the base of the rib cage. Through these two electrodes flows a constant current of 4 mA at 100 kHz. The other two terminals are located at the base of the neck and at the level of the xyphosternal junction and serve as voltage probes.

2.1.2 Contactless EM systems

Detection of human physiological activity through contactless EM systems is based on the recognition of displacements of a reflecting surface, and this is possible because both respiratory acts and heart beating modify fundamental parameters (frequency, phase, amplitude, and time of flight) of an EM wave reflected by the human body.

Frequency modulation is appreciable only when measured motions produce phase variations $d\phi/dt$ comparable to the frequency of the impinging microwave, which is not the case for relatively slow physiological activities like breathing or heartbeat.

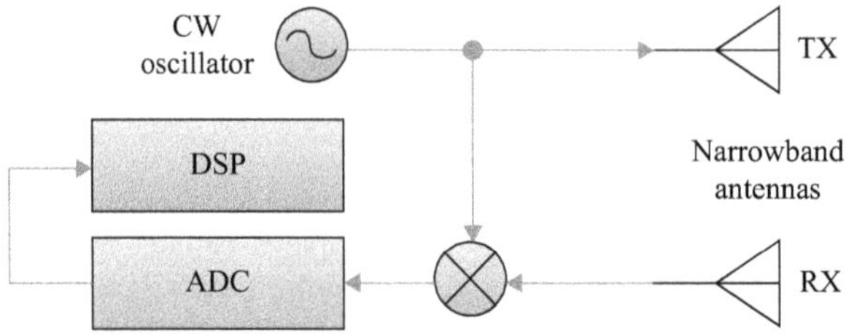

Figure 2.2 Block diagram of a CW Doppler radar with baseband demodulation

Also amplitude changes due to path loss variations are negligible for small movements, typically in the order of millimetres.

Therefore only phase and arrival time changes can be used for the detection of movements and, as a consequence, Doppler radars and UWB systems are employed to retrieve these two parameters respectively.

Doppler systems for detection of vital signs are based on the transmission of a signal toward a target region and on the analysis of the phase changes of the reflected waves, revealing target movements.

Transmissions are generally based on a Continuous Wave (CW), and phase variations, caused by the displacement of the reflecting surface, are proportional to both the wave frequency and the displacement itself. As a result of the narrow system bandwidth and modest analog-to-digital conversion speed requirements, Doppler radars are also suitable for compact designs and low-cost systems for medical applications. Figure 2.2 shows a basic block diagram of a CW Doppler radar, while in [27] different architectures are reviewed.

The idea for revealing thorax movements remotely using microwave radar techniques starts as early as the 1970s. In a pioneering work of 1976, C.I. Franks compares different methods and describes a radar which has been used to record, during 24 h, the respiratory activity of a newborn [28]. This paper already reveals a drawback of the phase-shift detection method of the stationary wave: a distortion of the measured signal depending on the mean position of the moving surface, which enhances high order harmonics at the expense of the fundamental.

Some years later a Doppler radar operating at the frequency of 24 GHz for the monitoring of artery wall movements associated with the pressure pulse waves [29] is presented. In [30] a system is proposed for detecting the physiological status of wounded human subjects, describing the circuit and performance for a 10 GHz wave, also with the use of a simplified theoretical EM model of the moving surface representing the human chest.

Other interesting contributions can be found in [31,32] where aspects related to the digital processing of the received signals are analysed and several techniques to make the processing more robust are described and implemented.

Recently a remarkable implementation has been presented [33], which is able to detect both pulmonary and cardiac motions at 50 cm. This work shows also some

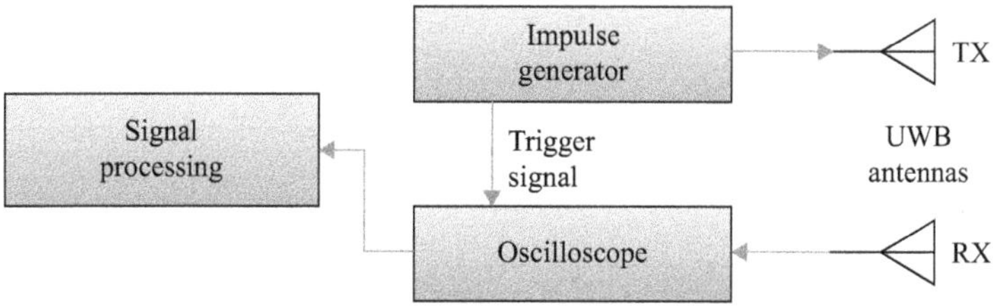

Figure 2.3 Block diagram of a UWB radar system

valuable considerations regarding the signal calibration to compensate for imbalance factors of the measurement chain.

According to [34], UWB systems have several key advantages over CW radars: the pulse has a wide frequency spectrum that can easily pass through obstacles, the pulse duration is very small (in the order of nanoseconds) and it allows a very high resolution. The short pulse leads to a low energy consumption, good immunity against multipath interference and allows both detection and positioning of a human being. In [35] a novel algorithm is proposed for detection of periodic motion caused by respiratory acts of trapped victims under rubble for low signal-to-noise-and-clutter ratio conditions. Since UWB systems rely on the measurement of the time of flight (TOF) of a pulsed wave [36,37], their only drawback is the need for a suitable hardware for pulse shaping in the transmitting subsystem and for very fast detectors in the receiving section, which leads to an increased cost if compared to Doppler systems (Figure 2.3). They are also able to eliminate the interfering pulses due to reflections of unwanted targets, but again this needs a fast switching discriminator to enable the receiver for the required time window and in this case the distance of the target must be known *a priori* [38].

In this book chapter an EM system based on the use of frequency sweeps over a wide band is presented, which can be considered as a trade-off between the CW and the UWB methods. Main features of both techniques can be joined and the disadvantages overcome.

A time–frequency matrix can be built storing the backscattered field sweep values in a time window. In this way data stored in each row carry information about the reflected signal in the RF frequency domain at a certain time, whereas data in each column represent the time evolution of that signal at a particular frequency. It is like having multiple CW measurements at the same time, therefore it is possible to average out the frequencies that contribute with erratic fundamental harmonic. The same data allow to retrieve the subject's distance like a UWB radar is able to do, yet having a much simpler (and cost-effective) hardware realization.

The next section shows the main theoretical backgrounds and the original results, which have allowed to develop an algorithm for determining both the fundamental frequency of an oscillating reflecting surface, such as a human chest during breathing, and its distance from the antenna, without the need of a UWB pulsed signal, and still avoiding sensitivity issues that affect Doppler systems at unpredictable frequencies.

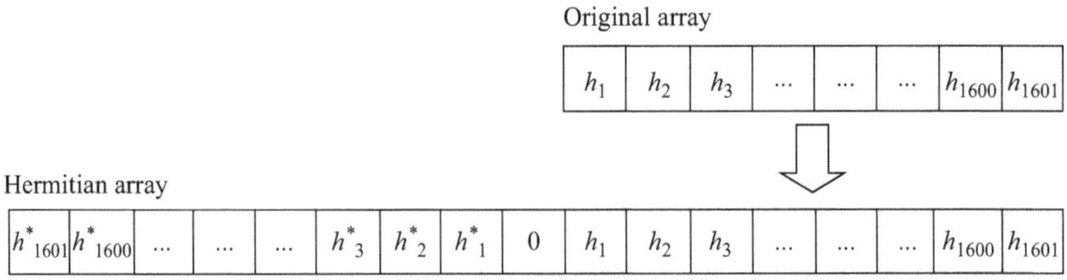

Figure 2.4 Example of how the new vector with Hermitian symmetry is obtained

2.2 Contactless breathing monitoring

2.2.1 Physical principle

The first studies were carried out by examining the EM scattering reflection coefficient S_{11} of a metal plate (i.e. a highly reflecting surface) placed at slightly different positions from the antenna, to investigate the impact of a reflecting surface, which will later be the human chest/belly, on this parameter.

Preliminary results were obtained at first using a Vector Network Analyzer (VNA) set to operate in the range from 3.74 MHz to 5.98 GHz. This has allowed to retrieve a vector of 1601 S_{11} values in this range with a uniform spacing ($\Delta F = 3.74$ MHz). A previously measured vector of a backdrop measurement (i.e., without reflecting surface) has been subtracted to this vector to purge the array from the antenna constant reflection coefficient.

The knowledge of a sequence of reflection coefficients measured at a certain time but at different frequencies allows to determine the distance of the obstacle from the emitting antenna, just like a UWB radar would through the computation of TOF.

To obtain a radar signal in time domain, starting from frequency data acquired by measurements, a technique borrowed from digital signal processing theory has been adopted [39,40]. To this purpose, we have built a new array which contains both the values returned by the instrument and their complex conjugate (flipped from $-F_{max}$ to $-F_{min}$) to have a complete spectrum including negative frequencies. The only missing value is the one at 0 Hz which has been considered as 0, since it only affects the mean value of the inverse transform. This operation can be made easily as we chose the ΔF equal to F_{min}. Figure 2.4 explains how the vector with Hermitian symmetry is obtained. Computing the inverse transform of the resulting array, using a standard IFFT algorithm, a time domain (or space domain) signal is achieved. As an example, for the spectrum obtained with the still obstacle placed at 3.23 m the graph shown in Figure 2.5 is obtained.

Finally, an evaluation of the best frequency range able to give proper results without using such a large bandwidth has been made. In fact, the wider is the band, the harder is to design the antenna and the hardware of the circuit.

Since the pulse obtained using an inverse transform of a reduced range of 3–5 GHz range is quite clean and symmetrical, and such a band is adequately free

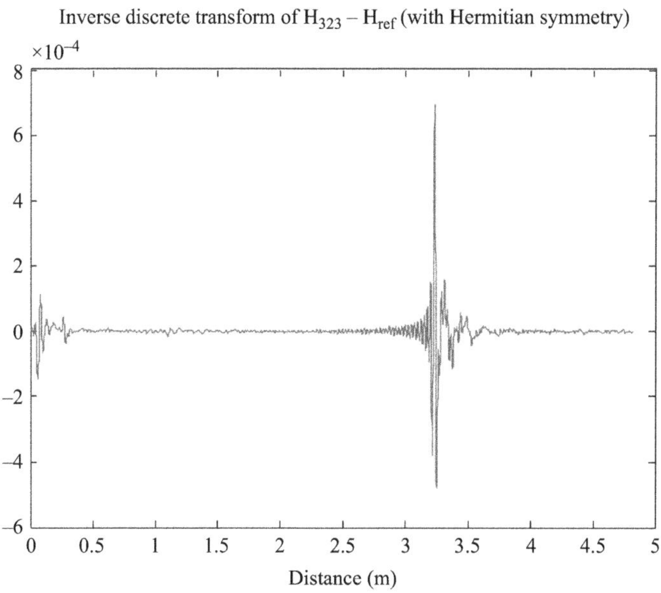

Figure 2.5 Inverse transform of the vector obtained with the obstacle placed at 3.23 m after subtracting the backdrop measurement

from communication systems,[1] we have decided to consider this range as a design requirement for the antenna and the hardware.

Further theoretical studies were made to determine the relationship between the periodical motion of an obstacle in front of the antenna (which has a certain set of harmonic coefficients), with the harmonic coefficients of the S_{11} signal that is measured by the VNA. The setup consists of an antenna that radiates an EM wave toward a scattering object at a distance l, considering any other unwanted reflections suppressed. By considering the scattering parameter S_{11} at the port of an Rx/Tx well-matched antenna as

$$S_{11}(F) = \Gamma(F)e^{j(4\pi F/c)l} \tag{2.1}$$

and assuming that the obstacle is placed in the far-field region, with the dislocation range $\pm\delta$ much smaller than the distance l_0, and also assuming as a first step that the obstacle is moving according to a sinusoidal law at a normalized angular frequency $\omega = 2\pi f = 1$, it is possible to define the motion as:

$$l(t) = l_0 + \delta \sin(t) \tag{2.2}$$

[1]Standard IEEE 802.11y-2008 allows Wireless LAN (WLAN) channels both at 3.6 GHz and 4.9 GHz but they are licensed in the United States only. Regarding WLAN 5, European standard EN 301 893 (current version v1.8.1) covers 5.150–5.725 GHz operation.

which yields to a time-varying S_{11}:

$$S_{11}(F,t) = \Gamma(F)\mathrm{e}^{2j\beta l(t)} = \Gamma \mathrm{e}^{j\tau_{l_0}F}\mathrm{e}^{j\tau_\delta F \sin(t)} \tag{2.3}$$

having defined each $\tau_x = (4\pi x/c)$. The complex coefficient Γ is not time-dependent due to the assumption $\delta \ll l_0$.

In order to evaluate the low-frequency harmonic content of S_{11}, we determine its Fourier coefficients:

$$\begin{aligned} A_n &= \frac{1}{2\pi}\int_{-\pi}^{\pi} S_{11}(F,t)\mathrm{e}^{-jnt}dt \\ &= \frac{\Gamma \mathrm{e}^{j\tau_{l0}F}}{2\pi}\int_{-\pi}^{\pi} \mathrm{e}^{-j[nt-\tau_\delta F sin(t)]}dt = \Gamma J_n(\tau_\delta F)\mathrm{e}^{j\tau_{l0}F} \end{aligned} \tag{2.4}$$

where $J_n(x)$ is the Bessel function of the first kind of order n. As expected, similarly to a phase modulated signal, the harmonic content of S_{11} caused by a sinusoidal moving reflecting object is composed of infinite harmonics whose amplitudes are related to the nth Bessel function of the first kind, and to a phase term depending on the frequency and the mean distance of the object. This simple result highlights that the choice of the working frequency F is a critical point. In particular, for any frequency F that satisfies

$$F_k = \frac{\bar{x}_{1,k}}{\tau_\delta} \tag{2.5}$$

where $\bar{x}_{1,k}$ is the kth zero of first-order Bessel function, the fundamental harmonic at ω cannot be detected with a CW signal because $J_1(\tau_\delta F_k) = 0$.

A more general result for Eq. (2.4) can be obtained for a generic moving object whose periodic displacement can be expanded in a Fourier series:

$$l(t) = l_0 + \sum_{k=1}^{\infty} \delta_k \sin(kt + \varphi_k) \tag{2.6}$$

for which it results:

$$A_n = \Gamma \mathrm{e}^{j\tau_{l_0}F} \cdot \mathop{\circledast}_{k=1}^{\infty} J_{\cdot,k}(\tau_{\delta_k}F, \varphi_k)|_n \tag{2.7}$$

where $J_{n,k}(c,\varphi)$ is an *extended* definition of the Bessel function:

$$J_{n,k}(c,\varphi) = \begin{cases} J_{n/k}(c)\mathrm{e}^{j(n/k)\varphi} & \text{if } n/k \text{ is an integer number} \\ 0 & \text{otherwise} \end{cases} \tag{2.8}$$

and the asterisk symbol is used to indicate the discrete convolution product of numerical sequences.

Expression (2.7) means that except for a phase shift term due to the mean value of the function (mean distance of the reflecting object) all the other terms are generated by the convolution of all Bessel functions produced by each harmonic. This dependence of the blind frequencies on the components of the motion of the backscattered signal makes the prediction of the best working frequency impossible.

2.2.2 Determination of target distance and respiratory rate

By stacking the arrays returned by the VNA, the result of storing the measurements of M sweeps, from time t_0 to t_{M-1}, yields a complex matrix H of size Mx$(N+1)$ whose rows are the M sweep vectors h and whose columns are time samples of S_{11}, measured at each of the frequencies from $F_{\min}$ to $F_{\max}$:

$$h_{i,k} = S_{11}(F_k)|_{t_i}\ , \text{ where } k = 0,\ldots,N, F_0 = F_{\min}, F_N = F_{\max} \tag{2.9}$$

$$H = [h_{i,k}] = [S_{11}(F_k)|_{t_i}] = \begin{bmatrix} S_{11}(F_0)|_{t_0} & S_{11}(F_1)|_{t_0} & \cdots & S_{11}(F_N)|_{t_0} \\ S_{11}(F_0)|_{t_1} & S_{11}(F_1)|_{t_1} & \cdots & S_{11}(F_N)|_{t_1} \\ \vdots & \vdots & & \vdots \\ S_{11}(F_0)|_{t_{M-1}} & S_{11}(F_1)|_{t_{M-1}} & \cdots & S_{11}(F_N)|_{t_{M-1}} \end{bmatrix} \tag{2.10}$$

As shown in the previous section, to avoid the results that are submerged by the antenna reflection coefficient and static clutter, and to better enhance differential displacements from a reference situation, a subtraction can be operated with a backdrop measurement. Or, missing a backdrop measurement, one of the samples can be subtracted, which could be the first acquired sample (for causality and online analysis) or a fixed row r of H, if data are stored for offline processing. But again for online analysis such a reference should be periodically re-instantiated for drift compensation and to take into account for changes in the position inside the room of moveable and reflecting objects like chairs, bottles, etc. This last solution proves to be much more effective since the contribution of the antenna is completely cancelled. An element of the differential matrix is then:

$$\bar{h}_{i,k} = S_{11}(F_k)|_{t_i} - S_{11}(F_k)|_{t_r} \text{ and } r \text{ is a fixed value} \in [0; M-1]. \tag{2.11}$$

To verify the feasibility of detecting the distance of a reflecting obstacle and measuring the fundamental frequency of its periodical distance variations, a series of tests has been performed using the VNA connected to the double ridge horn antenna and interfaced with a cable to a PC which stores and analyses the results. After the preliminary tests made using the metal plate, further tests involved the determination of the breathing frequency of a subject placed in front of the antenna. In this case the chest and belly of the subject represent the periodically moving obstacle.

Reported results refer to measurements made in an anechoic space, but additional experiments were carried out in home environments and in conditions with high reflective walls, with positive outcomes. The VNA has been set up to perform frequency sweeps in $N+1=71$ uniformly spaced points in 2 GHz-wide ranges (namely 1–3 and 3–5 GHz) at a power of 0 dBm.

By operating the inverse transform, after zero padding and Hermitian symmetry, for each row of measurement, it is possible to obtain a matrix of temporal displacements D which is represented in Figure 2.6 for the case of a subject breathing at 3.23 m in front of the antenna. In this figure a subtraction with the first measured array has been operated (instead of an no-human backdrop measurement) and the VNA was set

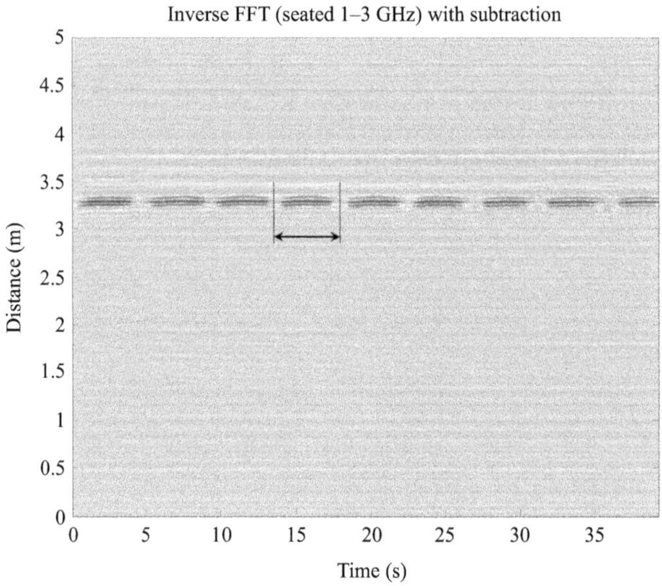

Figure 2.6 Surface plot of matrix of relative displacements over 40 s of measurements of a male subject seated at 3.23 m from the antenna. Arrows highlight a period of a respiration act

to scan the 1–3 GHz range. The average sampling period was 380 ms. The second test concerns the determination of the breathing frequency of a subject placed in front of the antenna.

From Figure 2.6, which basically represents a radar trace, it is possible to clearly distinguish a periodical pattern consistent with the breathing frequency of the monitored subject. Therefore the respiratory rate could be obtained by evaluating the temporal distance between two similar clusters in that graphic (arrows in Figure 2.6), e.g. analysing peaks of the autocorrelation function. Unfortunately, due to the high granularity of sampling and in case of non-ideal conditions where the clutter of the room strongly increases the noise on the graph, it would lead to a coarse approximation. A better estimate of the breathing frequency can be obtained in the frequency domain.

To evaluate the harmonic content of a complex time function $q(t)$ sampled at discrete times t_i, we can use the Approximate Fourier Transform (AFT) computed as a Riemann integration of the Fourier integral:

$$Q^{AFT}(f) = \sum_{i=0}^{M} q(t_i) \cdot \mathrm{e}^{-2\pi j f t_i} \cdot \Delta t_i \tag{2.12}$$

which, in case of uniform sampling (i.e. $\Delta t_i = \Delta t,\ t_i = i\Delta t$), corresponds to the discrete time Fourier transform (DTFT). The literature contains definitions both with and without the scaling factor Δt, which, in the second case, leads to a DTFT definition dimensionally equal to the sequence being transformed [39].

Therefore, the column-wise harmonic content of the H matrix can be evaluated as

$$H_k^{AFT}(f) = \sum_{i=0}^{M} h_{i,k} e^{-2\pi j f t_i} \Delta t \tag{2.13}$$

where $k = 0, \ldots, N$ is the index of the column, $\tilde{h}_{i,k}$ refers to each column purged from any bias, and the range of breathing frequency f (a continuous variable) is chosen to be from 0.05 Hz to $1/(2\Delta t)$, according to Nyquist–Shannon theorem.

The values are obtained by subtracting any linear trend present in the time window, to discard DC and other LF components that may be erratically detected by the FT algorithm caused by slow changes of position of the body and/or drifts on the measured data.

The average respiratory rate in a healthy adult at rest is usually given as 18–22 breaths per minute (0.3–0.37 Hz) [40] but it may vary widely according to the age of the subject, his general health conditions and kinds of physical activities made prior to the measurement session. On the other hand, the average acquisition rate Δt (about 380 ms) is much slower than the sweep time, due to data communication protocol, limiting the maximum detectable respiration rate without aliasing to 1.3 Hz, which however has proved to be enough during our tests.

The first two graphs of Figure 2.7 compare the AFT of two columns of the H matrix, for the case 1–3 GHz for 40 s, showing that column $k = 54$ (corresponding to 2.543 GHz) does not correctly detect respiration frequency, it rather shows the second- and third-order harmonics. The nearby column $k = 59$ (at 2.686 GHz) on the other hand properly shows a fundamental peak at 0.23 Hz, which is the real average breathing rate during the measured time window of 40 s; however, in this case the second-order harmonic is not detected, while the third is. This is the experimental evidence of the theoretical aspects previously discussed: the presence of blind frequencies that do not allow to retrieve the fundamental respiration frequency or some of its harmonics. Both this consideration and the experimental results show then that the blind frequencies are not so sparse, as implied by (2.5), and that even in a 2-GHz band there may be more than one frequency which does not correctly detect the fundamental. Since it is not possible to foresee which column provides the best spectrum, an averaging procedure has been applied. The magnitude of the resulting mean breathing spectrum as a real function of frequency f can be in fact computed as:

$$M(f) = \frac{1}{N+1} \sum_{k=0}^{N} \left| H_k^{AFT}(f) \right| \tag{2.14}$$

This is possible because each column contains harmonic information of the same phenomenon as seen from a different EM frequency, therefore despite the more or less sensitivity of each scanned frequency, the average spectrum is a better estimate of the global harmonic content. The spectral density obtained with (2.14) is shown in Figure 2.7(c): the fundamental frequency at 0.23 Hz correctly stands out as also higher order harmonics.

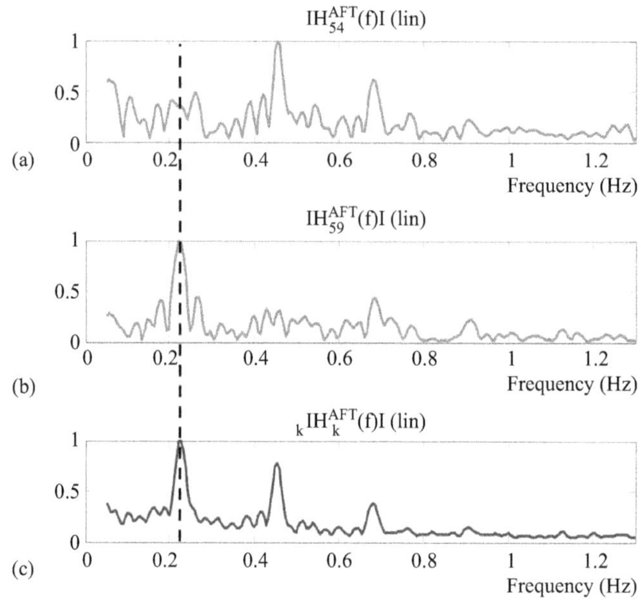

Figure 2.7 AFT of columns of H matrix (magnitudes only, normalized). Distance 3.23 m, sweep from 1 GHz to 3 GHz in 71 points, subject seated. (a) AFT of column $k = 54$; (b) AFT of column $k = 59$. (c) Sum of magnitudes of all columns using (2.14), normalized after sum

2.2.3 Offline and online application

To ease the storage for offline analysis of the data collected with both with EM instrumentation and reference measurement using an extensometric belt, a few MATLAB programmes have been implemented. One interfaces with the VNA and allows the recording of a certain number of samples (i.e. S_{11} sweeps). It is possible to define both the start and end frequencies of the sweep as well as the number of points in the chosen frequency range.

Concurrent measurements (i.e., EM system with the belt) were made by starting the acquisition manually at the same moment, because no common trigger signal was available in hardware. This could lead to some lag between measurements if signals are compared in time domain, but it has very low influence when comparing the spectra over an interval of 30 s or more.

Once the accuracy of the system has been assessed, as next sections will show, an online version of the same software has been made. This demo application displays the computed value of breathing frequency as the S_{11} data are retrieved from the instrument.

The working principle of the program relies on the theory explained in previous paragraphs. The main difference is that now instead of having a static H-matrix which has been stored previously, the matrix has a FIFO organization, where the

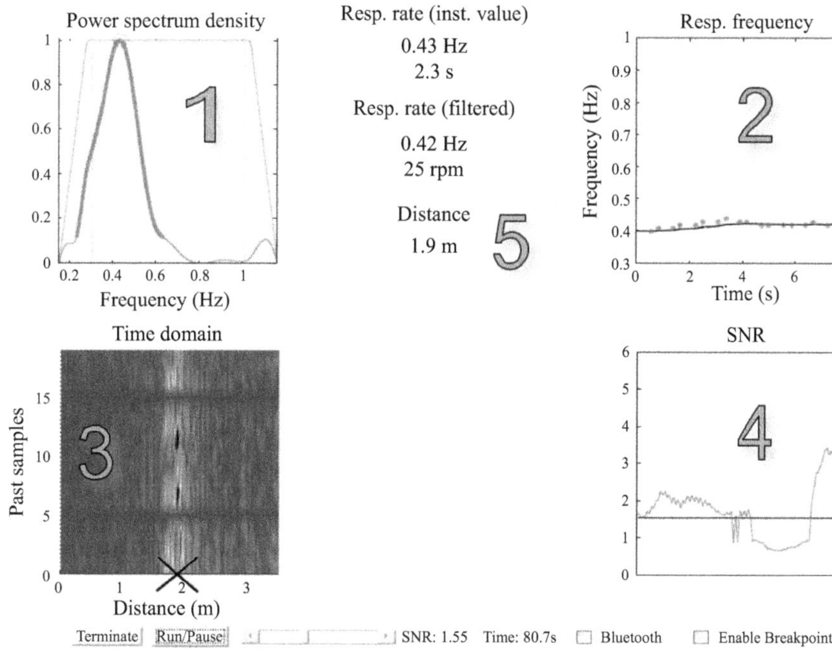

Figure 2.8 Screenshot of the online program

new array coming from the instrument enters the bottom and the oldest one leaves from the top. Each row can be used to evaluate the distance of the subject as seen in previous sections, while the average of the column-wise transforms is used to obtain an instantaneous spectrum, which is however obtained through a window, therefore a delay is always present. The window size is in fact a trade-off between accuracy and delay: a shorter window reduces the delay in case of sudden changes of respiration rate (like an apnoea event), but the main lobe gets larger and it doesn't resembles a peak anymore. On the other hand a wider window introduces too much delay even if it has the advantage of a narrow main peak.

Next Figure 2.8 shows a screenshot of the online application. It displays four graphs and some numerical values:

- On the upper left it is shown the current AFT obtained using (2.14) on the current window. Such a use of the transform on a moving window is often referred to as Short Time Fourier Transform (STFT) [17]. The circle locates the normalized maximum of the graph. The bold line represents the points around the peak which are therefore considered the "good part of the graph". The single-width line on the contrary are the points considered as noise, and therefore they should be as low as possible.
- The upper right graph shows the instantaneous frequency of the peak and past values up to 8 s (points indicate the exact values, while the line is a low-pass filtered value).

- The bottom left graph is the radar representation, like the one shown in Figure 2.2 but now time is in the vertical axis (the unit shown is the number of samples in the past, relative to present one). The peak (whose horizontal coordinate is the distance) is identified with a cross.
- The bottom right graph is the signal-to-noise ratio (SNR) which is computed as the ratio of the peak (ordinate of the circle in the first graph) to the value obtained averaging all the returned AFT values that are away from the peak (single width line in the first graph):

$$SNR = \frac{V_{peak}}{\langle V_{off-peak} \rangle} \tag{2.15}$$

  It is a slightly modified form with respect to the one used by Watanabe *et al.* [15], already cited in Section 2.1.1, where at denominator the second-order harmonic peak is also disregarded. The slider that is present at the bottom of the window allows to set the threshold (the horizontal line in last graph).
- The numbers in the middle top of the window show numerically the detected frequency in Hertz and period (seconds) of the instantaneous value, then below is displayed the frequency in Hertz and respiratory rate (in respiration acts per minute) of the filtered value. On the system monitor the numbers will be shown green if the SNR value is above the threshold and red if not (meaning that the value given may be not reliable). Finally it is shown the distance as detected by the red cross of the bottom left graph.

2.2.4 Experimental results

After the preliminary tests, an extended campaign of measurements has been undertaken to compare the results with those obtained from other reference devices, such as:

- The piezoelectric belt: ADInstruments MLT1132 (sensitivity: 4.5 mV/mm)
- The laser beam distance meter: MEL M25L/20 (10 mm range, 6 m of resolution and 25 kHz of bandwidth)
- The spirometer: ADInstruments ML311 with MLT1000L

Analogical data coming from these instruments were acquired at a sample speed of 1 kHz using the Data Acquisition ADInstruments 4/25T and its standard software LabChart 7. The experimental setup is shown in Figure 2.9.

Preliminary tests were made in the anechoic space of our laboratory using the Double Ridge antenna. After the design of the custom wideband antenna has been completed, more comparison tests between the two antennas in cluttered environments of our department, like rooms characterized by walls realized with plastic modular panels and containing office furniture were made. Additionally, more realistic tests have also been performed in different rooms of a real home with concrete walls, as it will be shown in the next section. The first trial set of measurements involved two target persons, a man and a woman. The data from the laser meter, belt, and the EM system were acquired. The spirometer was employed in place of the belt only for a subset of 10 measurements. The positions of the subjects were: seated in front of the

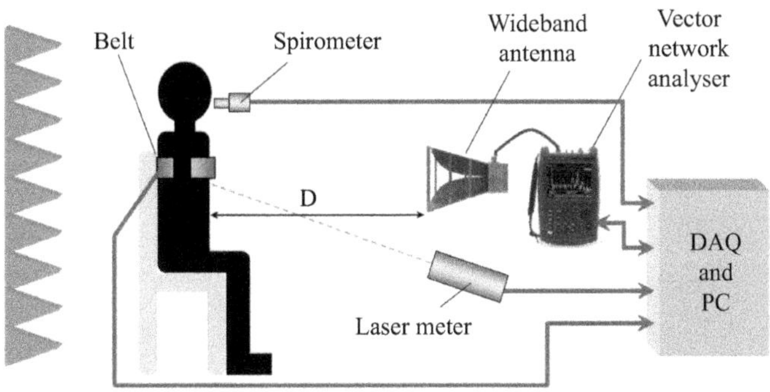

Figure 2.9 Experimental setup

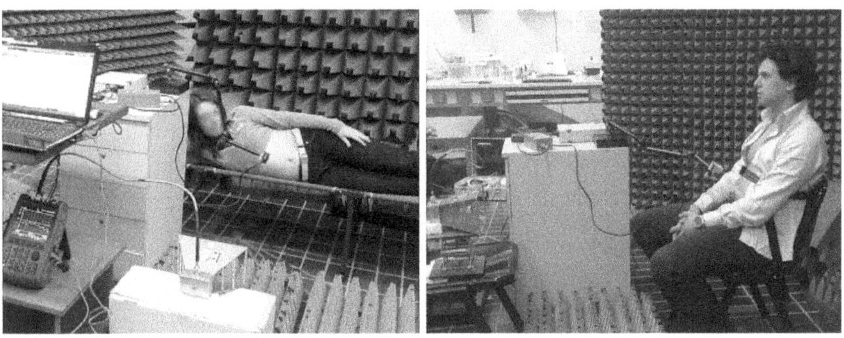

Figure 2.10 Example of two tests. The woman (left) is laying on her side. The antenna is visible in the foreground. The man (right) is seated and wears the belt

antenna standing tall in front of the antenna and laying on side on a crib (so that the chest was facing the antenna). Figure 2.10 shows a couple of pictures taken during the tests.

Finally, three kinds of breathing rate were measured: normal, forced fast, forced slow. The antenna was placed at 1.1 m from the zone of the body between the chest and belly of the subject and the scan range was from 1 to 6 GHz in 176 points; power was set at 0 dBm.

Figure 2.11 shows a screenshot of the offline program that analyses data and allows to compare the detected fundamental frequencies of breathing. On the left it is possible to choose the dataset, while the other graphs show the time evolutions of the laser signal and the belt/spirometer (when available). Below each time signal is represented the magnitude of their Approximate Fourier Transform obtained according to (2.12), therefore the unit of the vertical axis is coherent with that formula. For the EM system no time sequence is shown but only the average AFT obtained according to (2.14).

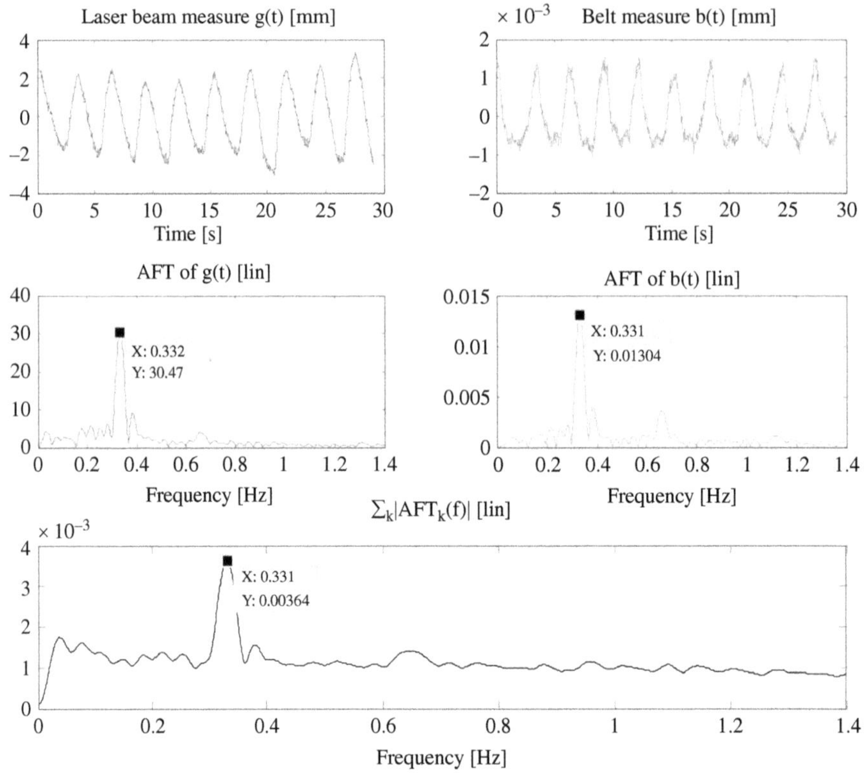

Figure 2.11 The algorithm compares the peak positions returned by: laser beam, respiratory belt and EM system measurements. The figures show an example of comparison, concerned a specific scenario: woman, seated, normal breathing, duration 30 s, trial 3 of 5. The x-coordinate [Hz] highlighted for each graphs is the respiration frequency detected by relative system

Figure 2.12 reports a table with all the combinations of measurements and the average results. It can be seen that for all the tests the mean difference between the EM system and the laser meter or the belt is less than 2 mHz. Anyway, as highlighted in the orange cells, there are some results that have a very high standard deviation caused by some noisy measurements in one of the three systems (EM, laser, or belt).

2.3 Prototype realisation

The results shown in previous sections pave the way for a possible application of the remote monitoring of breathing activity. By realizing a system that implements only the required subset of functions of a VNA, the resulting device may be installed inside

No. of Meas.	Duration (s)	Subject: Male	Subject: Female	Instrumentation: EM	Instrumentation: Laser	Instrumentation: Belt	Instrumentation: Spir.	Position: Seated	Position: Standing	Position: Laying	Breath rate: Normal	Breath rate: Slow	Breath rate: Fast	Mean Err w/Laser (mHz)	Std Dev w/Laser (mHz)	Mean Err w/Belt (mHz)	Std Dev w/Belt (mHz)
10	60		■	■	■			■			■			–0.1	1.37	–	–
5	30		■	■	■	■		■			■			0.0	1.00	0.0	1.22
5	30		■	■	■	■		■				■		0.8	0.45	1.8	1.30
5	30		■	■	■	■		■					■	0.4	1.82	0.6	1.14
10	60		■	■	■		■	■			■			–0.3	1.64	–0.4*	1.51*
9	60		■	■	■	■			■		■			–0.4	1.33	–1.5	3.96
2	30		■	■	■	■			■		■			–4.0	2.83	–8.5	10.61
4	30		■	■	■	■			■			■		–2.5	25.46	–21.8	51.18
2	30		■	■	■	■			■				■	–2.5	0.71	–31.0	18.38
5	30		■	■	■					■	■			–1.0	2.12	–	–
5	30		■	■	■					■		■		0.6	3.65	–	–
4	30		■	■	■					■			■	1.8	3.40	–	–
5	30	■		■	■	■		■			■			–1.4	8.26	1.0	2.12
5	30	■		■	■	■		■				■		2.4	1.52	2.6	3.78
4	30	■		■	■	■		■					■	–0.3	9.25	0.7	7.27
5	30	■		■	■	■			■		■			–0.8	18.51	1.0	17.03
2	30	■		■	■	■			■			■		7.5	4.95	9.3	8.91
5	30	■		■	■	■			■				■	5.4	23.38	4.0	21.44
5	30	■		■	■					■	■			1.8	1.64	–	–
5	30	■		■	■					■		■		1.6	0.89	–	–
5	30	■		■	■					■			■	–1.0	2.35	–	–
													Weighted mean error and std. dev:	**0.32**	**7.96**	**–1.57**	**15.52**

*This result pertains to the spirometer.

Figure 2.12 Measurement plan and test results

a home without compromising end user privacy and may be hidden into the wall or ceiling behind optically opaque plastic enclosures, thus having low impact on the appearance of the rooms.

The aim of this section is to present the realised sensing system, the results on the performance of the custom antenna and to explore the capability of the system to provide additional information from the backscattered signal, such as the subject's position and motion/activity inside a room.

2.3.1 Ambient assisted living and the HDomo 2.0 Project

The Ambient Assisted Living (AAL) is a term coined in the early 2000s to describe a set of technology solutions designed to make active, intelligent, and cooperative the environment we live in, making it capable to support independent living, to provide more security, simplicity, well-being and satisfaction in the performance of activities of daily living.

The main goals declared by the European AAL Association are [41,42]:

- Help maintain the health and functional capacity of elder people;
- Promote better lifestyles and more health for people at risk;
- Extend the period in which people can live in their preferred environment, by increasing their autonomy, self-sufficiency and mobility;
- Increase safety, prevent social exclusion and maintain a network of relationships of people;
- Support workers, family members and organizations in the assistive field;
- Improve the efficiency and productivity of resources in the ageing society.

Of course AAL is not just about the design of new and smart technologies, because it also requires in all its stage, from concept to implementation and use, the cooperation and effective communication between researchers, planners, industry, users, social and health workers.

Towards this aim the research developed in this work can be considered a contribution to the first three points listed above. In modern and rich countries, the expenditure for the health care is continuously rising, mainly for the increasing of population age. This happens specifically in European countries where the health care is prevalently public. In particular, in Italy most of the regions spend more than 70% of their budget in health care and the reduction of this expenditure without the reduction of the level of assistance is a key challenge at present. In this background, Marche Region has recently issued calls for projects aimed to design systems to be used in home automation for elderly care, providing an effective support for the prevention of accidents as well as for early detection of the typical health problems of the elder. In 2013, the Marche Government financed the HDomo 2.0 project, with the objective of creating systems which can provide basic information on the health status and habits of elderly people in their home, and devices that can help them in their everyday life. All these devices are supposed to be integrated into one system that can be easily installed at home and can be willingly accepted by elder persons since its main purpose is to have low invasiveness. In the context of this project, starting from the results explained in previous section, an ad hoc antenna and an electronic data acquisition system for the monitoring of breathing have been realized.

2.3.2 Wideband antenna

After the preliminary experiments carried out using the double ridge antenna, a smaller antenna, easier to handle and to install, has been realized during the project [43]. The antenna includes also a containing box behaving as a reflector (dimensions: $10 \times 10 \times 5.5$ cm) whose main purpose is twofold: increasing the directivity and decoupling the antenna from the rear wall where it will be installed. The design requirements of the antenna were its size, which should have been as small as possible, and its bandwidth which has been chosen in the range of 3–5 GHz as previously said.

After a first design stage made with the aid of a commercial software, the antenna has been realized and tested. The antenna has the required bandwidth and good directivity (from 8 to 10 dBi within the bandwidth with a halfbeam angular width of 46° over H-plane). At first, the system was tested inside a controlled environment in our laboratory, then it was tested in a concrete house. In order to verify the accuracy of the measurements, the respiration belt was used as a reference

2.3.2.1 Tests in laboratory

The first test is a comparison of system performances obtained using the double ridge antenna (bulky and heavy) and the new antenna (small and lightweight) both in the anechoic space and in a real environment. The setup involves a woman volunteer who is seated at 3 m from the antenna. Each measurement is made in the 3–5 GHz range, with a radiated power of 0 dBm, recording both the belt and EM data. The volunteer has been asked to breath normally, slowly and quickly. For each configuration three recordings of 60 s were taken. Figure 2.13 shows the detailed results, where we can see that basically there is no difference in sensitivity between the two antennas.

	Antenna		Breathing speed			Meas. 1			Meas. 2			Meas. 3		
	Double ridge	Custom	Norm.	Slow	Fast	EM (mHz)	Belt (mHz)	Δ%	EM (mHz)	Belt (mHz)	Δ%	EM (mHz)	Belt (mHz)	Δ%
In the anechoic angle	■		■			331	331	0.0%	329	329	0.0%	324	332	−2.4%
	■			■		171	171	0.0%	171	168	1.8%	170	169	0.6%
	■				■	800	800	0.0%	794	797	−0.4%	652	690	−5.5%
		■	■			331	332	−0.3%	338	337	0.3%	342	344	−0.6%
		■		■		147	149	−1.3%	170	170	0.0%	173	173	0.0%
		■			■	798	801	−0.4%	800	803	−0.4%	795	803	−1.0%
Outside the anechoic angle	■		■			330	334	−1.2%	327	331	−1.2%	333	334	−0.3%
	■			■		168	167	0.6%	163	164	−0.6%	171	168	1.8%
	■				■	799	802	−0.4%	799	803	−0.5%	798	802	−0.5%
		■	■			334	336	−0.6%	330	331	−0.3%	330	336	−1.8%
		■		■		166	165	0.6%	165	167	−1.2%	161	162	−0.6%
		■			■	795	800	−0.6%	810	814	−0.5%	796	800	−0.5%

Figure 2.13 Comparison of the double ridge antenna and the custom one

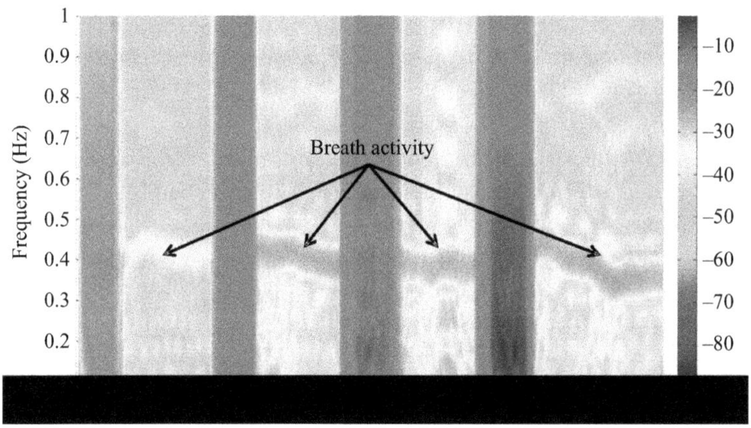

Figure 2.14 Breathing frequency is detectable despite of the environment. The vertical stripes represents the transients caused by the position changes of the subject

A second test regards the capability of detection of breathing frequency regardless of the static clutter. Since the algorithm averages the contributions at all EM frequencies and filters only the motions, the spectrogram in Figure 2.14 shows that the breathing activity (at about 0.4 Hz) is always detectable in all four different conditions, from left to right:

- The subject is seated in the anechoic space at 3 m from the antenna aperture;
- Same as the above but the subject has moved closer, at 1.8 m;
- The subject has moved outside the anechoic space, at 2.5 m from the antenna, towards a spot of the laboratory with office furniture;
- The subject has moved at 2 m with a metal surface at his back.

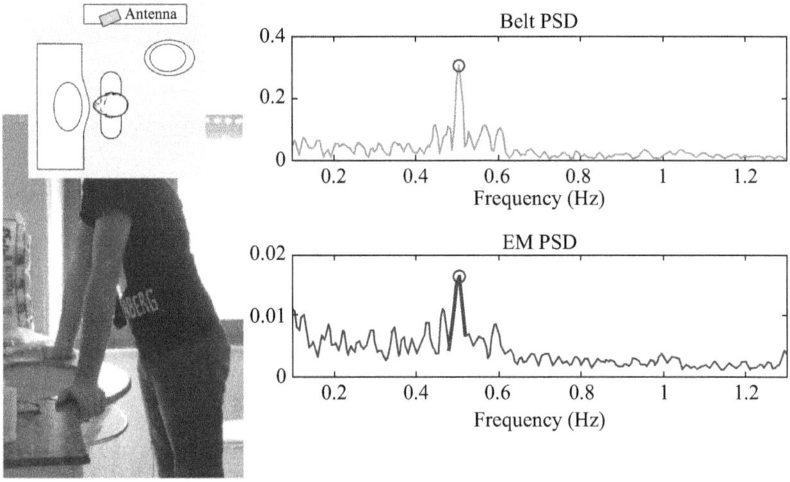

Figure 2.15 Comparison of Belt and EM PSDs for a measurement in the toilet

The vertical stripes are the transients that are caused by the change of position of the subject and/or of the measuring setup (which has been placed on a trolley in the middle of the room and rotated towards different directions inside the laboratory). Despite the change of the environment, above all for the last setup which involved a highly reflective surface, the breathing activity can always be detected as the region with the highest intensity within each rest area.

2.3.2.2 Tests at home

A campaign of 118 measurements was conducted inside a standard Italian house (concrete walls). They were made in three different environments: lounge, toilet, and bedroom. All the measurements present good accuracy, but for the sake of brevity only the most significant ones are reported, while more outcomes can be found in [44]. First interesting results are about a fast breathing measurement made on a male volunteer standing in front of the washbasin of the toilet. The custom antenna was placed on the windowsill at 1.32 m and was facing the side of the man (but rotated a little bit), practically at the height of the pelvis. Yet as shown in Figure 2.15 (the antenna is hidden behind the body of the volunteer), the EM systems return a result very similar to the one of the belt.

Other measurements have been made in the lounge, where a female volunteer was seated on a couch located to the side of the room, while the antenna was located on a shelf near the TV set at about 1.6 m. This time the result is very poor because of the position of the subject which is too much lateral with regard to the radiation diagram of the antenna (indicated by the arrow in Figure 2.16), even if her chest was at the same height.

The results obtained in these two different situations are important in terms of correct antenna placement inside a real house: if the subject is placed inside

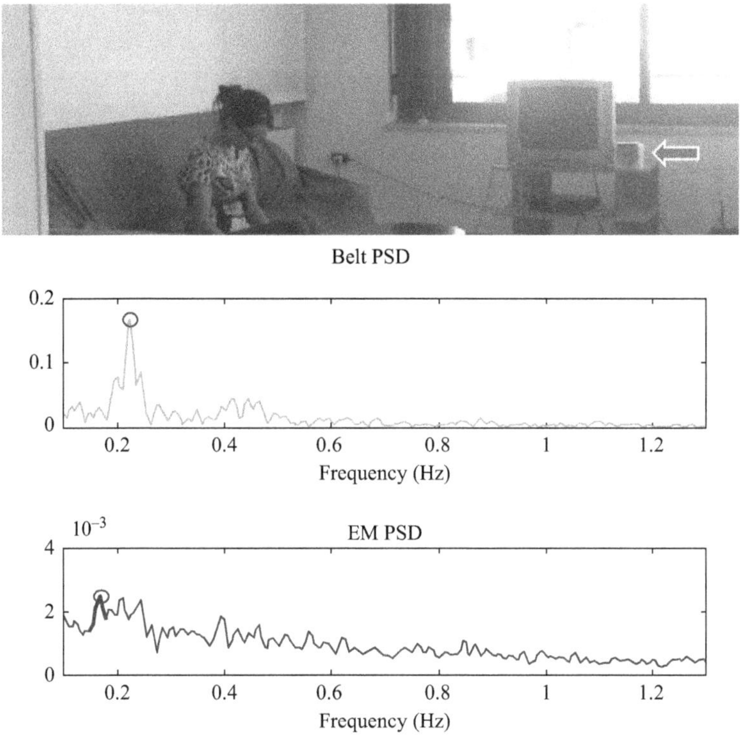

Figure 2.16 Comparison of Belt and EM PSDs for a measurement in the lounge

the main lobe of the antenna, whatever his/her position is (side or even back), a good result is always obtained. This is because closeness and multiple reflections, caused by furniture and walls, strengthen the harmonic content that is detected. On the other hand, if the subject is too far and/or outside the main lobe of the antenna it would be more difficult to pick the correct component. Other tests demonstrated that the system is able to detect the distance of the subject from the source. Figure 2.17 (top) shows the radar diagram of a one-minute recording of a subject breathing on the couch. The bottom figure shows the sum of the absolute values of all the inverse transforms and its envelope. The antenna is located in front of the user at 3 m of distance. Of course, despite the backdrop subtraction the result is noisier with respect to the one that would be obtained in a controlled environment, as demonstrated by the spurious peaks at about 2 m and at around 1 m. These are caused by spatial aliasing of multiple paths caused by the rear wall and ceiling that are folded in the region of interest. In other words these are echoes that could be located at a longer distance by reducing the interval of the sweep. Therefore the number of points of the frequency range is a parameter that must be designed according to the dimensions of the room where the system is installed, to allow that only the main desired reflection enters the monitored range.

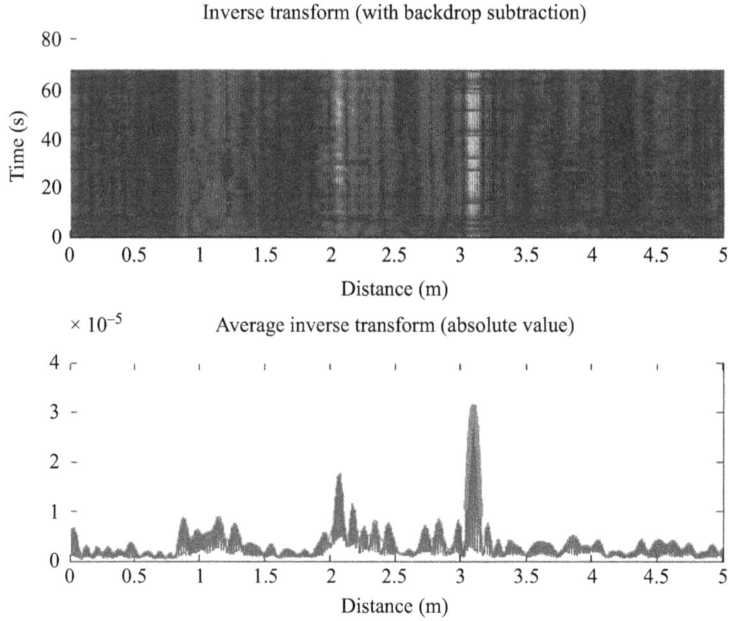

Figure 2.17 Inverse transform of one minute of breathing on the couch. (Top) Radar diagram; (bottom) average of absolute values of radar diagram

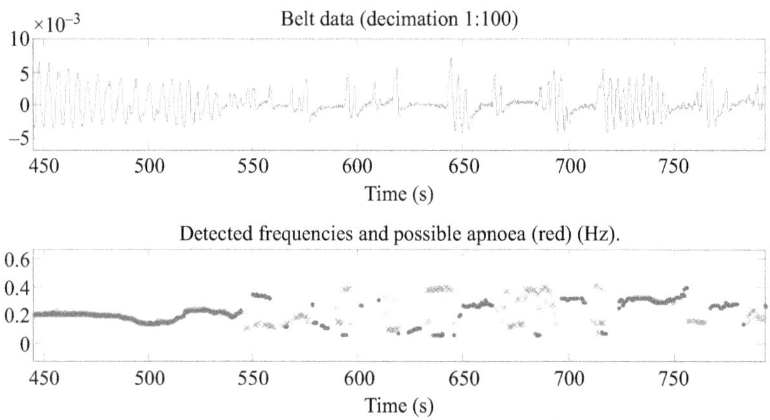

Figure 2.18 Zoomed portion of short sleep monitoring. When the EM signal becomes too weak, unreliable data are marked with cross

Finally, a comparison of the respiratory rate detection between the belt and the EM system (using the custom antenna and the VNA) on a non-stationary test is shown. In this experiment, a 50-min nap on bed is recorded. Figure 2.18 shows a small portion (about 5 min) of the complete log, where from the belt data are clearly

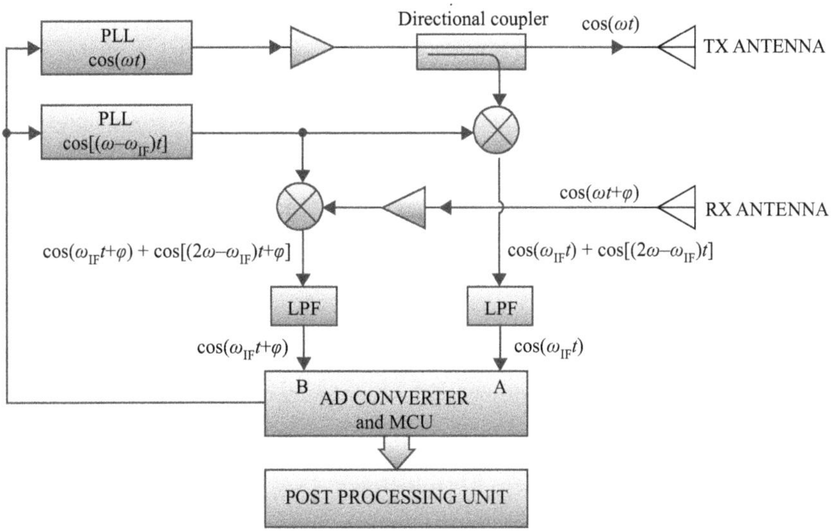

Figure 2.19 Block diagram of the prototype TX/RX unit for HDomo 2.0 Project

identifiable the apnoea episodes, highlighted in yellow. Before the signal becomes too weak the two detection systems provide same values which therefore are overlapped (i.e. frequencies detected using belt data and EM data, respectively). Then, when the signal becomes too weak, the algorithm recognizes that EM computed frequency values have a too small SN ratio and a too low average spectrum, therefore marks some of the subsequent values as "unreliable readings", which occur in correspondence with apnoeas. The overlapping is again present when breathing returns temporarily regular.

2.3.3 Hardware implementation

The physical implementation of the system has been discussed and planned with the industrial partners of HDomo 2.0 project. In particular:

- R.i.co. Srl (Castelfidardo) for the HW design and SW coding;
- SSG Srl (Fabriano) for the routing of the raw data provided by the system through a gateway;
- Apra Spa (Jesi) for the gathering, handling and display of the collected data.

The final block diagram of the realized device is shown in Figure 2.19. It basically traces the TX/RX structure of a VNA when measuring the S_{21} with two ports. This solution has been preferred since it has been seen that using single antenna and a directional coupler exposes to the following drawbacks.

- An external directional coupler commercially available is bulky and very expensive, which is not advisable for a product that is intended for mass production. In practice about 80% of the cost of the system will be covered by this component alone.

- A directional coupler designed directly on the printed circuit board on the other hand has no cost, but it would be extremely sensible to the PCB production process.
- In both cases the coupling factor for the reflected signal is very low on the needed frequency range, meaning that the reflected signal, which is already weak on its own, is even more attenuated. Therefore it must be strongly amplified before entering the processing unit, radically worsening the SNR.

The proposed solution on other hand has the only drawback that the system is bulkier and it must be taken care to decouple the antennas to prevent that the transmitted signal enters directly into the RX channel.

The core of operations is made by a microcontroller. The designers at R.i.co. have chosen the STM32F303RCT6 which is an ARM-based Cortex-M4 processor.

Two external PLLs (LTC6948) are used to set the transmitted frequency and the demodulating frequency. These devices allow the generation of RF frequencies up to 6.39 GHz with a resolution of 38 Hz, therefore they can be used to generate the desired frequency sweeps with a significant granularity.

The MCU sets the parameters of these PLLs via two Serial Peripheral Interfaces (SPI). When operating at a single frequency, one PLL is programmed to generate a certain frequency F that is output from one antenna and the other is set at slightly lower frequency ($F - F_{IF}$) where the Intermediate Frequency (IF) is $F_{IF} = 500$ kHz. One mixer performs a multiplication between these two signals obtaining two components: one at about double frequency and one at the intermediate frequency. After a low pass filter only the IF signal is sampled, which will be used as a reference (Input A in Figure 2.19).

Coming from the RX antenna of Figure 2.19 a phase-shifted signal is present, which is again multiplied by the second PLL, returning, after the low pass filter, a second signal that keeps the same phase shift (Input B) and can be compared to the reference. Since the micro-controller has the capability to sample at 5 MSps, it is then possible to obtain 10 samples per period for each wave. By changing the frequency F and keeping constant the intermediate frequency it is possible to use a frequency-independent algorithm to detect the amplitude and phase shift of the two sampled signals.

Figure 2.20 shows the realized prototype where the main components are highlighted. The emitted power is 11 dBm and it allows to determine the breathing frequency in the anechoic space up to 4 m.

2.3.4 Software implementation

The first release of the code works only at a single frequency and more efforts must be done to perform a frequency sweep. In particular, as a next step, the settling time required for the PLLs to switch from one frequency to another has to be studied, since this duration strongly influences the capacity of performing a frequency sweep in a short time. The entire operation of sampling and computing the vectors from 128 samples on both channels (A and B) requires 25.5 ms. Every four computations, the average vector is evaluated and output on the serial port. For this reason, the

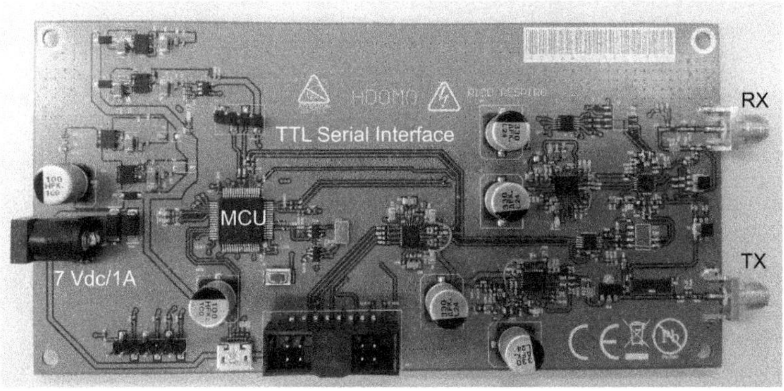

Figure 2.20 Prototype of the TX/RX board and main components

system produces a complex value proportional to the required S_{11} every 102 ms. The computation of vectors A and B whose amplitude and phase relationship can be conformed to an S_{11} measurement is:

$$A = \sum_{n=1}^{128} x_n \cdot e^{-2j\pi(F_{IF}/F_s)n} \quad B = \sum_{n=1}^{128} y_n \cdot e^{-2j\pi(F_{IF}/F_s)n} \tag{2.16}$$

where x_n and y_n are the detrended samples taken from the reference ADC and the reflected signal ADC respectively (Figure 2.19). Therefore an estimate of the S_{11} at the output frequency F is:

$$\bar{S}_{11} = g(F)\frac{B}{A} \tag{2.17}$$

where the complex coefficient g is frequency-dependent and takes into account that the ratio may have magnitude greater than one since the two signals go through different amplification stages before being compared, therefore such a parameter should be calibrated so that the final result is one when the transmitted and received signals are exactly the same. The C language implementation of such a simple code did not require a library for handling complex numbers and it has been easily made using standard trigonometric functions.

The RF board finally outputs a couple of numeric values (magnitude of B/A ratio and phase difference in degrees) every 102 ms on a standard 115200,N,8,1 serial port (TTL). Preliminary checks were made by simply connecting a serial TTL-to-USB converter to a PC to analyse data. The data proved to be reliable, therefore the final realization of a standalone prototype has involved, as the post-processing unit, the use of an embedded Linux system for the transform computation and data display. This latter part was not strictly required by the project however it has been implemented for debug and demonstration purposes. The final commercial device may be re-conceived with the only computational unit and gateway interface with no display.

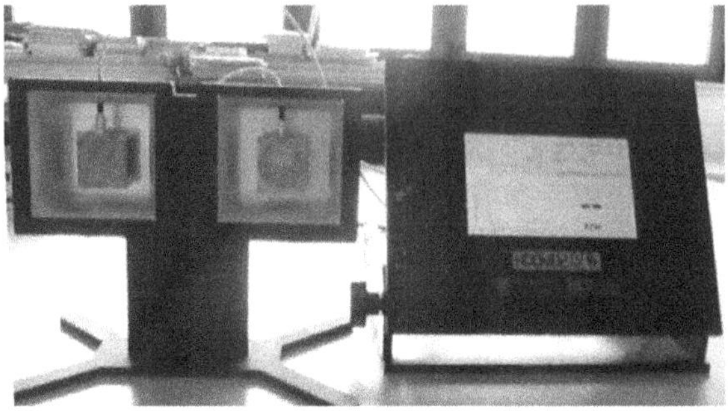

Figure 2.21 Stand-alone real-time device working at a single frequency

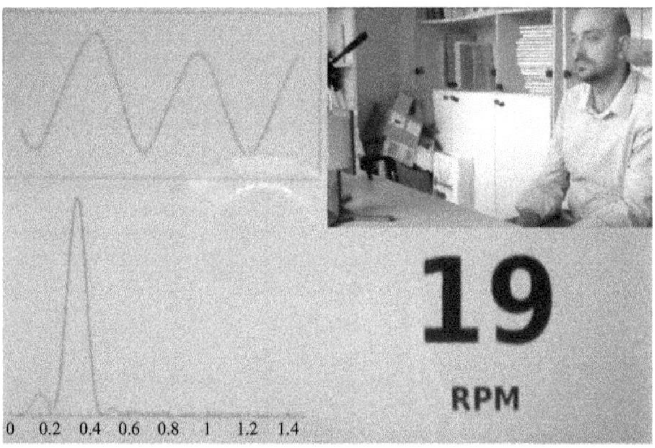

Figure 2.22 Frame of the demonstration video showing the display of the system. In the upper left it is visible the phase of the signal and below its AFT in the range of 0–1.4 Hz

Figure 2.21 shows the final boxed device: the TX/RX antennas are on the left, while the touch-screen display of the Linux system is on the right. In Figure 2.22 the details of the screen is reported: this is a screenshot of a demonstration video where it is shown how various breathing situations (normal breathing, fast breathing and apnoea) are detected by the system, therefore it is possible to compare the result (expressed in Respiratory acts Per Minutes) with the other overlay video in the upper right which shows the actual breathing.

2.4 Conclusions

In this chapter it has been shown that by using a frequency sweep technique to record, for each frequency, the phase shift between the reflected and emitted waves, it is possible to detect the breathing frequency of a subject. This demonstrates that to achieve such a result is not necessarily required for the complex hardware normally used when implementing a UWB radar, but, since the proposed system performs many CW analysis in parallel, a design similar to a CW architecture is suitable.

More in details, it has been mathematically and experimentally demonstrated that a CW system may fail in detecting the fundamental frequency of a moving surface and therefore the proposed method can be considered more robust, yet keeping the hardware complexity reasonably low.

Moreover, the advantages of EM waves on other methods have been pointed out, since their contactless nature leads to no privacy issues and no concerns about clothes or other dielectric materials interposed between the antenna and the subject.

Results have been validated both in a controlled environment and in a real house with concrete walls. The proposed system uses a 2 GHz bandwidth signal, therefore a custom antenna has been designed and realized. Although the best results are obtained when the subject is in front of the radiating element, acceptable outcomes were collected even in disadvantageous conditions, like when the subject is located with his side facing the antenna, while more attention must be paid if he is located on a side lobe of the radiation pattern.

Within the regional project HDomo 2.0 a prototype of the TX/RX board and the processing unit has been built. Even if the RF circuit has the full capability of performing a frequency sweep, its current implementation works at a single frequency. Future developments involve the realization of a suitable code on the prototype for testing the frequency sweep function and the validation of the results on a clinical trial setup.

References

[1] P. Rashidi and A. Mihailidis, "A survey on ambient-assisted living tools for older adults," *IEEE Journal of Biomedical and Health Informatics*, vol. 3, no. 17, pp. 579–590, Nov. 2013.

[2] L. Scalise, V. Mariani Primiani, P. Russo, A. De Leo, D. Shahu, and G. Cerri, "Wireless sensing for the respiratory activity of human beings: measurements and wide-band numerical analysis," *International Journal of Antennas and Propagation*, vol. 2013, Article ID 396459, 10 pp, 2013.

[3] P. Marchionni, L. Scalise, I. Ercoli, and E. P. Tomasini, "An optical measurement method for the simultaneous assessment of respiration and heart rates in preterm infants," *Review of Scientific Instrumentation*, vol. 84, no 12, pp. 121705, 2013.

[4] G. Capelli, C. Bollati, and G. Giuliani, "Non-contact monitoring of heart beat using optical laser diode vibrocardiography," in *2011 International Workshop on BioPhotonics*, Parma, Italy, June 2011, pp. 1–3.

[5] L. Boccanfuso and J. M. O'Kane, "Remote measurement of breathing rate in real time using a high precision, single-point infrared temperature sensor," in *2012 Fourth IEEE RAS EMBS International Conference on Biomedical Robotics and Biomechatronics (BioRob)*, June 2012, pp. 1704–1709.

[6] I. Sato and M. Nakajima, "Non-contact breath motion monitor ing system in full automation," in *2005 IEEE Engineering in Medicine and Biology 27th Annual Conference*, 2005, pp. 3448–3451.
[7] S. D. Min, D. J. Yoon, S. Yoon, and M. Lee, *A Study on a Non-contacting Respiration Signal Monitoring System Using Doppler Ultrasound*. Berlin, Heidelberg: Springer Berlin Heidelberg, 2007, pp. 864–867. [Online]. Available: http://dx. doi.org/10.1007/978-3-540-36841-0_207
[8] S. D. Min, J. K. Kim, H. S. Shin, Y. H. Yun, C. K. Lee, and M. Lee, "Noncontact respiration rate measurement system using an ultrasonic proximity sensor," *IEEE Sensors Journal*, vol. 10, no. 11, pp. 1732–1739, Nov. 2010.
[9] P. Arlotto, M. Grimaldi, R. Naeck, and J.-M. Ginoux, "An ultrasonic contactless sensor for breathing monitoring," *Sensors*, vol. 14, no. 8, p. 15371, 2014.
[10] D. Rapoport, R. Norman, and M. Nielson, *Nasal Pressure Airflow Measurement*. Pro-Tech Services Inc. 2001, 2001.
[11] R. Norman, M. Ahmed, J. Walsleben, and D. Rapoport, "Detection of respiratory events during NPSG: nasal cannula/pressure sensor versus thermistor," *Sleep*, vol. 20, pp. 1175–1184, 1997.
[12] R. Budhiraja, J. Goodwin, S. Parthasarathy, and S. Quan, "Comparison of nasal pressure transducer and thermistor for detection of respiratory events during polysomnography in children," *Sleep*, vol. 28, pp. 1117–1121, 2005.
[13] C. Vaughn and P. Clemmons, "Piezoelectric belts as a method for measuring chest and abdominal movement for obstructive sleep apnea diagnosis," *Neurodiagnostic Journal*, vol. 52, pp. 275–280, Sep. 2012.
[14] A. Okken, *Recurrent Apnea in Newborn Infants*. O. Prakash, Springer Netherlands, vol. 10, no. 3, 1984.
[15] K. Watanabe, T. Watanabe, H. Watanabe, H. Ando, T. Ishikawa, and K. Kobayashi, "Noninvasive measurement of heartbeat, respiration, snoring and body movements of a subject in bed via a pneumatic method," *IEEE Transactions on Biomedical Engineering*, vol. 52, no. 12, pp. 2100–2107, Dec. 2005.
[16] P. Chow, G. Nagendra, J. Abisheganaden, and Y. T. Wang, "Respiratory monitoring using an air-mattress system," *Physiological Measurement*, vol. 21, no. 3, p. 345, 2000.
[17] W.-Y. Chang, C.-C. Huang, C.-C. Chen, C.-C. Chang, and C.-L. Yang, "Design of a novel flexible capacitive sensing mattress for monitoring sleeping respiratory," *Sensors*, vol. 14, no. 11, p. 22021, 2014. [Online]. Available: http://www.mdpi.com/1424-8220/14/11/22021
[18] T. Klap and Z. Shinar, "Using piezoelectric sensor for continuous-contact-free monitoring of heart and respiration rates in real-life hospital settings," in *Computing in Cardiology 2013*, Sep. 2013, pp. 671–674.
[19] T. Yoshimi, M. Ito, K. Yanai, T. Sato, T. Harada, and T. Mori, "Infant condition monitoring system and method using load cell sensor sheet," 28 August 2001, US Patent 6,280,392. [Online]. Available: https://www.google.com.ar/patents/US6280392

[20] Z. T. Beattie, C. C. Hagen, M. Pavel, and T. L. Hayes, "Classification of breathing events using load cells under the bed," in *2009 Annual International Conference of the IEEE Engineering in Medicine and Biology Society*, Sep. 2009, pp. 3921–3924.
[21] O. Polo, L. Brissaud, B. Sales, M. Besset, and A. Billiard, "The validity of the static charge sensitive bed in detecting obstructive sleep apnoeas," *European Respiratory Society Journal*, vol. 1, no. 4, pp. 330–336, 1998.
[22] E. Svanborg, H. Larsson, B. Carlsson-Nordlander, and R. Pirskanen, "A limited diagnostic investigation for obstructive sleep apnea syndrome: oximetry and static charge sensitive bed," *Chest*, vol. 98, no. 6, pp. 1341–1345, 1990.
[23] D. I. Townsend, M. Holtzman, R. Goubran, M. Frize, and F. Knoefel, "Measurement of torso movement with delay mapping using an unobtrusive pressure-sensor array," *IEEE Transactions on Instrumentation and Measurement*, vol. 60, no. 5, pp. 1751–1760, May 2011.
[24] K. Konno and J. Mead, "Measurement of the separate volume changes of rib cage and abdomen during breathing," *Journal of Applied Physiology*, vol. 22, no. 3, pp. 407–422, 1967. [Online]. Available: http://jap.physiology.org/content/22/3/407
[25] R. Seeton and A. Adler, "Sensitivity of a single coil electromagnetic sensor for non-contact monitoring of breathing," in *2008 30th Annual International Conference of the IEEE Engineering in Medicine and Biology Society*, Aug. 2008, pp. 518–521.
[26] A. Fein, R. F. Grossman, J. G. Jones, P. C. Goodman, and J. F. Murray, "Evaluation of transthoracic electrical impedance in the diagnosis of pulmonary edema." *Circulation*, vol. 60, no. 5, pp. 1156–1160, 1979.
[27] C. Li and J. Lin, "Recent advances in doppler radar sensors for pervasive healthcare monitoring," in *2010 Asia-Pacific Microwave Conference*, Dec. 2010, pp. 283–290.
[28] C. I. Franks, B. H. Brown, and D. M. Johnston, "Contactless respiration monitoring of infants," *Medical and Biological Engineering*, vol. 14, no. 3, pp. 306–312, 1976.
[29] J. Y. Lee and J. C. Lin, "A microcprocessor-based noninvasive arterial pulse wave analyzer," *IEEE Transactions on Biomedical Engineering*, vol. BME-32, no. 6, pp. 451–455, Jun. 1985.
[30] K. M. Chen, D. Misra, H. Wang, H. R. Chuang, and E. Postow, "An x-band microwave life-detection system," *IEEE Transactions on Biomedical Engineering*, vol. BME-33, no. 7, pp. 697–701, Jul. 1986.
[31] B. Lohman, O. Boric-Lubecke, V. M. Lubecke, P. W. Ong, and M. M. Sondhi, "A digital signal processor for doppler radar sensing of vital signs," *IEEE Engineering in Medicine and Biology Magazine*, vol. 21, no. 5, pp. 161–164, Sep. 2002.
[32] A. Droitcour, V. Lubecke, J. Lin, and O. Boric-Lubecke, "A microwave radio for doppler radar sensing of vital signs," in *2001 IEEE MTT-S International Microwave Symposium Digest*, vol. 1, May 2001, pp. 175–178.

[33] W. Hu, Z. Zhao, Y. Wang, H. Zhang, and F. Lin, "Noncontact accurate measurement of cardiopulmonary activity using a compact quadrature doppler radar sensor," *IEEE Transactions on Biomedical Engineering*, vol. 61, no. 3, pp. 725–735, Mar. 2014.
[34] A. G. Yarovoy, L. P. Ligthart, J. Matuzas, and B. Levitas, "UWB radar for human being detection [same as "UWB radar for human being detection", ibid., vol. 21, no. 11, 06]," *IEEE Aerospace and Electronic Systems Magazine*, vol. 23, no. 5, pp. 36–40, May 2008.
[35] A. Nezirovic, A. G. Yarovoy, and L. P. Ligthart, "Signal processing for improved detection of trapped victims using UWB radar," *IEEE Transactions on Geoscience and Remote Sensing*, vol. 48, no. 4, pp. 2005–2014, Apr. 2010.
[36] I. Y. Immoreev, S. Samkov, and T.-H. Tao, "Short-distance ultra wideband radars," *IEEE Aerospace and Electronic Systems Magazine*, vol. 20, no. 6, pp. 9–14, Jun. 2005.
[37] I. Immoreev and S. Ivashov, "Remote monitoring of human cardiorespiratory system parameters by radar and its applications," in *Fourth International Conference on Ultrawideband and Ultrashort Impulse Signals, 2008. UWBUSIS 2008*, Sep. 2008, pp. 34–38.
[38] D. Dei, G. Grazzini, G. Luzi, *et al.*, "Non-contact detection of breathing using a microwave sensor," *Sensors*, vol. 9, no. 4, p. 2574, 2009.
[39] F. Eng, F. Gunnarsson, and F. Gustafsson, "Frequency domain analysis of signals with stochastic sampling times," *IEEE Transactions on Signal Processing*, vol. 56, no. 7, pp. 3089–3099, Jul. 2008.
[40] G. J. Tortora and N. P. Anagnostakos, *Principles of Anatomy and Physiology*. New York, Harper-Collins, 1990.
[41] http://www.aal europe.eu, Tech. Rep., last accessed 23/01/2017.
[42] http://www.foritaal2012.unipr.it/ambient-assisted living, Tech. Rep., last accessed 23/01/2017.
[43] V. Di Mattia, V. Petrini, E. Pallotta, *et al.*, "Design and realization of a wideband antenna for non-contact respiration monitoring in AAL application," in *2014 IEEE/ASME 10th International Conference on Mechatronic and Embedded Systems and Applications (MESA)*, Sep. 2014, pp. 1–4.
[44] P. Russo, V. Petrini, L. Scalise, *et al.*, "Remote monitoring of breathing activity and position of a subject in indoor environment: the HDomo 2.0 project," Sep. 2015, pp. 19–22.

Chapter 3

Technology-based assistance of people with dementia: state of the art, open challenges, and future developments

Susanna Spinsante, Ennio Gambi, Laura Raffaeli, Laura Montanini, Luca Paciello, Roberta Bevilacqua, Carlos Chiatti, and Lorena Rossi

Abstract

The impact of dementia and other cognitive diseases on the capability of making everyday life activities is well-known, as well as it has been demonstrated that dementia may strongly affect not only the life of the person affected, but also the surrounding relatives. In fact, in the majority of the cases, the caregiver of a person with dementia is a family member, who usually loses the possibility to run a normal life, because of the burden of assistance. As a consequence, a number of research projects have been carried out, under the umbrella of different funding schemes, to identify the right technologies able to support caregivers of people with dementia, both informal and formal ones.

This chapter provides first a review of the research and market state of the art of assistive technologies for dementia. Then, from this analysis, the requirements, barriers and success factors of the different solutions are identified and discussed. Two projects are presented in detail, to cover the domain of technologies for informal caregivers, applied at home where the patient with dementia lives; and to show how similar technologies, in a different architectural arrangement and with the provision of different services and functionalities, may be used in nursing homes and care institutions. Conclusions regarding the current stage of development and open issues are finally presented in the last section.

3.1 Introduction

Based on the latest Diagnostic and Statistical Manual of Mental Disorders (DSM V) criteria [1], dementia is classified as a major neurocognitive disorder because it interferes with both cognitive function and performing everyday activities. Cognitive function refers to memory, speech, language, judgment, reasoning, planning and other thinking abilities. Examples of everyday activities are making a meal, paying bills and traveling to a store to make a purchase.

Alzheimer's Disease (AD) is the most common cause of dementia, which accounts for an estimated 60 to 80 percent of cases. Among the symptoms associated to AD, it is possible to mention: difficulty in remembering recent conversations, names or events, which is often an early clinical symptom; apathy and depression. Later symptoms include impaired communication, disorientation, confusion, poor judgment, behavior changes and, ultimately, difficulty speaking, swallowing and walking. Revised criteria and guidelines for diagnosing Alzheimer's were proposed and published in 2011: they recommend that AD be considered a slowly progressive brain disease that begins *well before* clinical symptoms emerge.

An estimated 5.4 million Americans of all ages have Alzheimer's disease in 2016. This number includes an estimated 5.2 million people aged 65 and older [2], and approximately 200,000 individuals under age 65 who have younger-onset Alzheimer's [3]. According to the estimations provided by the World Alzheimer Report 2015 [4], over 46 million people live with dementia worldwide, and this number is projected to increase to 131.5 million by 2050.

The situation is further exacerbated by the fact that AD affects not only the patients, but also their families or informal caregivers, on whom the main burden of care falls, putting them at higher risk of stress, anxiety, mortality and lower quality of life [5]. Caregiving for a person with dementia can lead to physical and psychological morbidity. Although depression, aggression and sleep disturbances are the most frequently identified patient's symptoms that impact negatively on caregivers, a wide range of symptoms are associated with caregiver burden and depression [6]. The psychological and behavioral symptoms of dementia, that are the most challenging ones for the informal caregivers, could be the ones that can be truly supported by technology, for example, with respect to monitoring the disease progression.

Technology-driven interventions hold the promise of convenient, low-cost methods of delivering psychosocial interventions. However, despite the positive findings confirmed in systematic reviews, like the one by Godwin *et al.* [7], evidence remains controversial concerning the effectiveness of providing support to caregivers of AD patients, through case management, counseling, training, technological devices and the integration of existing care services. A proposal of an effective assistive technology (AT) solution targeted to family and informal caregivers, as an alternative to, or a complementary form of, the care activities they deliver to AD patients, is still an open research area. Part of the difficulties and stress related to AD caregiving might be prevented by leveraging the potentials of new ICT solutions, and by developing innovative support services for AD patients. However, such solutions are not fully available in the market, and there is a general consensus that ICT potential is still far from being fully exploited. At the same time, promoting aging in place for AD patients should not represent a strategy to shift the burden of care from the formal services to the informal caregivers, with supervision constituting the largest proportion of the caring effort.

This chapter analyzes the different requirements for the design of technologies to assist caregivers of AD patients, which emerge from different application scenarios, and presents the results obtained from field experiments either about home-based AT adoption, and the use of AT in institutionalized care. A stronger focus is put on projects involving technical and scientific contributions from the coauthors. First, a project carried out as a multi-component randomized clinical trial (RCT), to reduce the burden of family caregivers of AD patients at home, is presented [8]. The trial focused on the design, prototyping and installation of an AT kit at each user's premise, to investigate the level of acceptance and the impact of the technological facilities on caregivers. The kit was designed to unobtrusively monitor AD patients at early stage, still able to stay at home, but needing to be assisted, usually by a relative or a caregiver. The technology solution used in the trial has been improved based on the feedback received from users, to provide a second, revised version, which is currently undergoing experimental evaluation in the field. Later on, a re-design and improvement of the same kit for use in a different scenario, i.e., assisted nursing homes, where needs and requirements are different from those pertaining to the private home scenario, was undertaken. The chapter reports the results obtained in all the different scenarios considered, which show some positive outcomes in facilitating the caring activities, both for informal and formal caregivers, but also highlights relevant issues to account for, related to the impact of technology on the AD patients, and on their daily routines.

3.2 State of the art

The large concern and demand by older persons to remain in familiar social living surroundings are stimulating many study projects joined with industries, especially across Europe, to improve health and wellbeing. While highlighting the latest updates in Europe and, in particular in Italy, regarding scientific projects dedicated to unraveling how diverse needs can be translated into an up-to-date technology innovation for the growing elder population, Lattanzio *et al.* in [9] also raise awareness about the indispensable role of geriatric medicine toward future guidelines on specific technology. In fact, AT shall be designed for those with specific geriatric-correlated conditions in familiar living settings, and for individuals aging actively, and technology developments are based on user needs identified by geriatricians.

3.2.1 Literature review

From the research conducted in the literature, it emerged a quite rich and large variety of issues discussed. In fact, advanced technology care innovation for older persons encompasses all sectors (AT, robotics [10], home automation, home care and institution-based healthcare monitoring, telemedicine) dedicated to promoting health and wellbeing in all types of living environments. Some studies focus on the types of technologies to be adopted for the assistance of people with dementia (PwD), others on the different aspects addressed by AT. Consequently, it is not possible to perform a unique classification of ATs, as it can be made depending on different features.

The aim of this subsection is to provide an overview of the researches carried out in the wide field of technologies for assistance of PwD.

The article by Maresova *et al.* [11] explores the modern information technologies which are currently used for the support and improvement of the quality of life of elderly people with dementia. It focuses on technologies for PwD especially connected with monitoring and communication: in addition to receiving information about the patients, ATs can also enable to contact them and give assistance for everyday activities, with the aim to reduce the effort of the caregivers. The support for everyday activities can include: providing verbal or pictorial instructions to perform an activity step by step, by means of a computer system connected to monitor sensors, or providing strategies for indoor orientation, by means of light indications that guide the person toward the destination.
Also the authors in [12] describe everyday technologies used for Alzheimer's disease (AD) patients' care, and classify them based on their purpose:

- monitoring technology;
- assistance technology;
- technologies for therapy;
- technology for diagnosis/assessment.

These technological solutions have different objectives, and intervene on different aspects of the care. Therefore, specific design and realization issues should be considered for each category.

Patterson *et al.* [13], instead, refer specifically to solutions for reminding a PwD to perform an activity. They state that even if there is much research on this problem, there is less focus on integrating reminding technology, adherence detection and reasoning, to create a self-management solution for dementia. They provide an overview of studies related to this issue and propose a prototype that aims at merging reminding technology with adherence detection, and communication with caregivers in case of non-adherence.

Another issue concerns what types of technologies can be adopted in the field of PwD's assistance. Some of the most common ones are cited in [14]:

- communication technologies, e.g., e-mail, real-time alarms, devices for telecare, social networking;
- robotics, which can provide help for household maintenance, or just perform companionship activities;
- home automation technologies, both for monitoring purpose and to ensure home safety features;
- sensors for monitoring, generating alarms and data collection. Common types of sensors are for example environmental (e.g., motion detection, presence, thermostats), radio-frequency transmitters for identification and computer-vision tools (e.g., for motion analysis).

The authors in [15] performed a research on currently available technologies for assisting PwD and caregivers, identifying the following fields of action: screening, memory-aid, monitoring health or safety, information sharing and telecare, communication support and therapy. All the solutions supporting these functions are helpful for the care of PwD, but caregivers can get more advantages if the data obtainable are stored and analyzed to infer behavioural patterns. The knowledge of behavioural patterns, in fact, enables caregivers to let PwD behave as they like, as long as no immediate risk is expected. Moreover, caregivers can minimize their interventions, if they can predict the consequences of particular actions.

ATs are helpful tools for both PwD and their caregivers, however some issues have to be investigated. First, in their review, the authors found that most of the studies focus on the technology development, but researchers have to consider the users' anxiety about it. Indeed, caregivers are worry about privacy violation, thus it could be useful to perform a large scale survey of the caregivers' needs in order to evaluate the technology acceptance. As for the care homes, an aspect often not evaluated is the architecture of the buildings, that should be designed in such a way that caregivers can watch over the patients. Finally, due to the increasing demand, care institutions need to recruit new workers, but, on the other hand, they have a limited budget. The high efficiency of care is also important, thus it is necessary to enable the caregivers acquiring and improving their skills.

Some attempts have been made to explore the use of so-called smart objects (SO) [16], with the purpose of monitoring well-being and supporting people's independent living. The study by Papetti *et al.* [17] tries to provide an overview of such products in order to understand if their features really match users' needs, and, consequently, if an environment embedded with SOs, like a smart home [18], can be considered as assistive too, taking into consideration the attributes given by the definition of the SOs, of being embedded in familiar objects and immerse in the users' surround.

The large variety of technologies addressed to different aspects of the care contributes to the possibility of personalizing the assistance. This is very important because each person with dementia shows different symptoms and has his/her own needs [14]. Caregivers provide the best assistance when they are able to interpret the patients' behavior and understand how to intervene [19].

3.2.2 Market analysis

The research on the state of the art showed a variety of solutions addressed to PwD, from single devices looking at specific aspects to more complex integrated systems, making use of both hardware and software products. Further, they can be categorized into solutions that act preventively, i.e., trying to predict potentially harmful incidents, and systems that detect either short-term emergencies (e.g., a fall) or long-term trends (e.g., changing of eating behaviours).

Emergency calling systems are among the most demanded solutions. There are commercially available products [20–22] consisting of a worn sensor equipped with a button to be pressed to call help. Other systems instead, do not require the user's intervention, for example [23] they use activity sensors to detect the absence of movement and provide warnings to the caregiver. One of the most dangerous emergency situations is represented by falls. Worn fall sensors have the disadvantage that could not be worn by the patient at the moment of the fall, thus different alternatives have been proposed [24–26] using detection methods such as video cameras, microphones or depth sensors like the Kinect. In this area, the research interest focuses also on fall prediction by means of gait analysis [27].

Another category of solutions available in the market deals with area access and navigational solutions, initially developed for professional care institutions working with PwDs. Indoor localization systems work with different technologies on the wireless LANs (WLANs), or adopt Radio Frequency Identification (RFID) and Bluetooth iBeacon [28,29]. On the other hand, outdoor solutions exploit the Global Positioning System (GPS) technology [30,31] (by means of both mobile apps and wearable devices like bracelets) to localize a missing person.

Research studies also focus on activity recognition and behaviour prediction, especially addressed to the detection of the so-called ADLs, i.e., Activities of Daily Living. This kind of approach is aimed at identifying the "normal" condition for the user, and consequently at detecting an abnormal situation that could suggest the need of intervention.

In the European and US markets, different products using monitoring principles have been introduced [32–34], which often integrate safety features and/or e-Health aspects.

The report in [35] contains a market overview of technology for aging in place. In this analysis, technologies are divided into different categories, and among those referred to dementia care, products related to engagement and location tracking are present. Likewise, from the study [36] conducted for the "Confidence" Project it emerged that currently there are different systems on the market addressing the orientation loss that often affects PwD. It is evident that these solutions are devised for people with mild dementia. For users in a more advanced state of dementia, on the other hand, it could be more useful to adopt a solution to monitor that the person does not exit from home.

With the aim to perform a mapping study for identification, analysis and classification of the existing ATs both in literature and in the UK market, the authors in [37] reviewed several works in this field. The first outcome is a classification of ATs into five main categories:

- robotics;
- health monitoring;
- prompts and reminders;
- communication;
- software.

The main functionalities covered are: activity monitoring, mobility (moving physically from a place to another), detection (abnormal behavior or changes from daily routine), cognitive help (for intellectual activities), health information, rehabilitation (especially for people with disabilities), socialization, leisure activities (like playing music, tourism, etc.). They found that even if the academic research mainly focuses on health monitoring and robotics, the UK industry develops health monitoring and software-based products, thus highlighting a partial gap between the two directions.

Such a list of features has been confirmed by the Alzheimer's society [38]. Therein, the authors present some categories of products designed to help people with Alzheimer's. Among them, the following ones stand out: reminders, medication aids, locator devices, communication aids, safety technologies, safer walking, telecare and devices to support social participation and leisure. Moreover, in this paper one of the main problems related to the adoption of assistive technology is highlighted: the cost. In fact, ATs can be very expensive, and the money spent on ATs does not represent a long-time investment in most of the cases, since the needs of an Alzheimer's patient, or more in general a person with dementia, change according to the disease progress. For this reason, a possible solution is to rent the AT only for the necessary period of time. In correlation to the high cost of ATs, from a study by Tegart *et al.* [39] emerged that the market demand is not sufficient, and operational implementations are not widespread. Consequently, assistive technologies are not a preferred option in healthcare delivery. This report refers to the Australian situation, and investigates barriers and success factors of assistive health technologies, that have influence on their large-scale adoption. The project highlighted the need for a sustainable business model; the development of the technology should be based on market needs and aligned with the expected outcomes. Moreover, the healthcare market is evolving, attracting new external players. The cooperation among interdisciplinary partners can contribute to the creation of integrated solutions and introduce a compelling suite of services on the market.

3.3 Requirements, barriers, success factors

Elderlies often feel insecure and frightened when testing technological solutions, so the trend in Ambient Assisted Living (AAL) projects is to put elderlies and their relatives at the center of the system design and development phases.

In this section, the requirements to consider in the design and development of a technological assistive solution are discussed, in addition to obstacles and success factors influencing their deployment, emerged from surveys and field studies.

The paper in [36] describes the results of a study for the collection of user requirements for electronic AAL products, obtained by following an iterative approach. It was conducted for the "Confidence" project, which aims at providing mobility and safeguarding assistance services adaptable on the personal needs of PwD. The idea in Confidence is to combine assistive technologies and personal help involving the social environment of PwD. During the first stages of the project, user requirements have been collected in three different countries (related to the partners involved in the project), and the results show that some needs are common to all the users, while others are country-specific, depending on factors such as the financial conditions, cultural aspects and public services. In all workshops and interviews, for each participating country, some general findings regarding the system acceptance emerged: country-specific requirements should be considered in order to achieve the system acceptance in each country; disease acceptance (both by patients and relatives) and patients' privacy protection are the most crucial requirements for the successful adoption of the system.

The reports in [40,41] summarize some outcomes of the research activities carried out within the project named "COMODAL", and reveal some insights into consumer and industry behaviour in the current marketplace of Assisted Living Technology (ALT). The study confirms the hypothesis that industry could better engage consumers with assistive technologies by better understanding their barriers and behaviour. From the literature study, it emerged that the main barriers to the markets for older consumers are:

- consumers do not perceive the need for assistive living products or services;
- consumers lack information or awareness of such products, services or solutions;
- consumers lack information on how or where to purchase, as well as they do not receive help and support in choosing the best product or service, in order to meet their needs and be cost-effective;
- there are differences in cultural views about the acceptability of assistive living solutions;
- concerns about privacy and control of health-monitoring services.

The "disconnection" between designers and consumers represents another barrier. The complexity of some products perceived by the users is often due to the fact that they are not designed following the users' needs and preferences. Moreover, in some cases there is a poor confidence or trust in the technology, a limited knowledge and training on how to use ALT, worries about maintenance and after-sale service.

In the framework of the same project, other surveys have been conducted with the aim to understanding the social and behavioral issues that discourage or encourage the purchase and use of ALT and e-ALT. Consumers and industry have similar views about which pre-purchase barriers affect the decision to buy or use these products, and that can be broadly ranked as: (a) cost; (b) information and awareness; (c) perception of the benefits of using products.

Even if there is a clear order in the influence power of the three aspects, they are rated differently by the two groups. In fact, it appears that industry overestimates the influence of other people's negative attitudes on consumers, and underestimates the influence of the cost of running a product, its complexity and user's feelings about information disclosure, reliability, design and safety of use.

On the other hand, the belief that a product would make daily living tasks easier, and the awareness that products/services exist to help people, are the most influential enablers for the purchase, and there is a greater synergy between both groups' views about these factors. Enablers have been rated as more influential than barriers, suggesting that positive messages about the benefits of using products would be very powerful and could provide greater assurances for consumers.

In Section 3.2, market studies on AT, referred to specific countries, were mentioned. These reports also include considerations about barriers and success factors. Many solutions do not go on after the pilot stage, due to several barriers that prevent their adoption [39]. By investigating the factors that have influence on the widespread adoption of ATs, economic, socio-cultural and technological barriers emerged. The main reasons are the lack of incentives, the non-knowledge of the potential benefits provided by the adoption of the technology, and the low availability of data to prove the business sustainability and cost effectiveness of the investment on AT.

Each type of technology can give rise to different problems, thus, for each category, specific design and realization issues should be considered.

Monitoring technologies can help PwD to prolong their independent living at home, and include for example devices for home safety and falls recognition. In this case, aspects to take into account include [12]:

- interference of the signals of wireless communication devices;
- the system is expensive to install and/or to monitor;
- hardware issues, such as: necessity to reset, sensors can be damaged, maintenance is needed;
- alert management: who has to send alerts to, and what situations cause alerts;
- data management: some monitoring technologies can generate huge amounts of data.

As for the AT, several solutions have been developed to support PwD for completing their activities of daily living, mainly addressed to provide prompts and step-by-step guidance. Some challenges for the design and implementation of these technologies include the following ones:

- integrate monitoring capabilities with the possibility to provide feedbacks to questions;
- modify technologies designed for a specific task in order to adapt to other tasks;
- work out what types of prompts to use and simplify the input methodology;
- monitor that the action prompted has been carried out, and foresee proper actions in case of non-compliance;
- manage system errors.

Technologies applied to cognitive training and reminiscence therapy instead have a different approach and entail other issues. First, the some of these technologies require a significant amount of time to design and develop. Secondly, they foresee interaction with participants, and their use require a certain level of expertise or familiarity with technology.

A common requirement emerging from the state-of-the-art analysis is the extreme importance of taking into account the profile of the AT user, as a basis to build the technological requirements of the intervention, and to reach a higher positive impact [42]. Through the User Centered Design (UCD), it is possible to draw up information on key concepts, such as attitude towards technology, acceptance and usability of any new products. The collected information serves for the technological development on one side, and for the Impact Assessment Analysis on the other one, that describes the future path of the devices. Bevilacqua *et al.* in [43] describe in details the most important metrics—attitude towards technology, usability and accessibility—for conducting a prompt evaluation of a new device for the older people, suggesting common guidelines and critical issues to solve.

3.4 Developed projects

3.4.1 Related studies

It has been observed that age-in-place has the potential to slow down the dementia progress and improve the PwD's quality of life [44]. To this aim, several ATs can be employed in order to help PwD living independently, such as smart homes, home environments equipped with a collection of software and hardware components enabling to monitor the resident person and understand their activities, as proposed in [45]. The authors apply a user-centered design following some key requirements of PwD: (a) new equipment needs to look like a previously seen and known one, and it should be first evaluated by caregivers; (b) PwD need to maintain a sense of control over their environment; (c) it is important to support caregivers by providing prompts and reminders.

Li *et al.* [46] propose an unobtrusive real-time system for supporting caregivers for the monitoring of PwD. It enables security management and abnormal situation management, considering four situations: the security feature includes fall detection, and detection of exit from a safe area, while, for the latter feature, the analysis of daily activity patterns and the sleep monitoring are performed. The operating mode is the following one: the sensor network (mainly wireless environmental sensors) acquires data that is processed by a server. The server sends data to a cloud model, in charge of storing and transferring information toward the registered mobile devices (i.e., to the caregivers). When a critical event is detected (fall or exit from a safe area), a warning is sent to the caregiver's mobile device. Moreover, daily activities and sleep are analyzed in order to obtain the baseline condition for the patient, and allowing to raise a warning in the case of abnormal behavior.

A monitoring system for dependent persons living alone at home or in a care facility is presented in [47]. The system adopts a multi-sensor network for presence monitoring, set up in the environment of the monitored person, in addition to a wireless identification system (RFID). The environmental sensors and the pressure detector in the bed are non-intrusive, and the presence sensors adopt infra-red technology, thus respecting the privacy of the users. The only wearable sensor is the miniaturized identification tag, embedded in clothing or worn on the body as a plaster. Thanks to an alarm system and a personalized behavioral analysis (which detects the activities and identifies a condition of normal behavior), the nurses are able to monitor the patients remotely through a web application, and also to intervene in case of dangerous situations. The application provides graphical representations about the trend of some features of interest: distance, motion speed, high agitation, group activity.

The system has been tested in an Alzheimer's care unit, involving only one patient and the caregivers, in order to demonstrate the possibility of deployment, then other validations should be performed. The markets to be explored for its deployment refer to specialized institutions, and non-independent people living at home.

Aloulou *et al.* [48] describe the development and deployment of an AAL system for nursing homes. It comprises a set of environmental sensors aimed at acquiring contextual information and monitoring the patient, a centralized machine for each room and devices for user interaction (to provide both reminders to patients and notifications to caregivers). The system trial involved eight patients with moderate dementia and their caregivers, in a nursing home in Singapore. Field trials are extremely important: in this case for example, the installation outside a laboratory environment led to identify problems emerging from the real usage. Secondly, the first test phase carried out only with caregivers enabled a preliminary evaluation of the system, and its improvement without affecting the patients. Finally, the complete test provided an overall description of the system capabilities, its effectiveness, the benefits brought to the patients and the caregivers, the contribution to improve the quality of the assistance provided and to support the caregivers.

The "Escort System" is another solution designed to be adopted in assisted living communities, to support the caregivers for the residents' monitoring. This case, however, only concentrates on the problem of wandering of PwD [49]. The purpose of the system is to identify the wandering events and to provide alarms to the caregivers, who can promptly intervene and prevent dangerous situations, such as falls. A low power wireless communication infrastructure is employed for indoor localization of the residents, who wear small badges. For each patient, different rules are defined that reflect potentially dangerous situations for him/her, and the alarms for the caregivers are generated according to these personal rules, in order to avoid a large number of unnecessary notifications.

3.4.2 UpTech, UpTech RSA, Tech Home

The authors of this chapter have been involved in three different projects dealing with the assistance of PwD that are described in the following subsections. Specifically, all these projects propose support tools for the patients' assistance, and are addressed to caregivers, either formal or informal.

The three solutions deal with the monitoring of people, but often this activity is seen as a violation of the users' privacy. For this reason, with the aim to respect privacy requirements and to provide unobtrusive monitoring, only simple environmental sensors have been employed, resulting less intrusive and more acceptable than other devices like wearables or video cameras.

3.4.2.1 UpTech

The UpTech project has already concluded, it involved PwD who can live in their homes but need assistance. Actually, the project was oriented to the family caregivers, who are often subjected to much stress due to the effort and the worry about the patients' safety. The main project objectives were to reduce the burden of the assistance for the caregivers, to maintain AD patients at their homes, and to improve the quality of life of all the users [8]. A group of nurses and social health operators performed periodical visits to the patients' houses to provide assistance. In addition, a technological kit was supplied and installed in the homes of a group of participants, with the aim to continuously monitor the safety of the patients. The choice of the

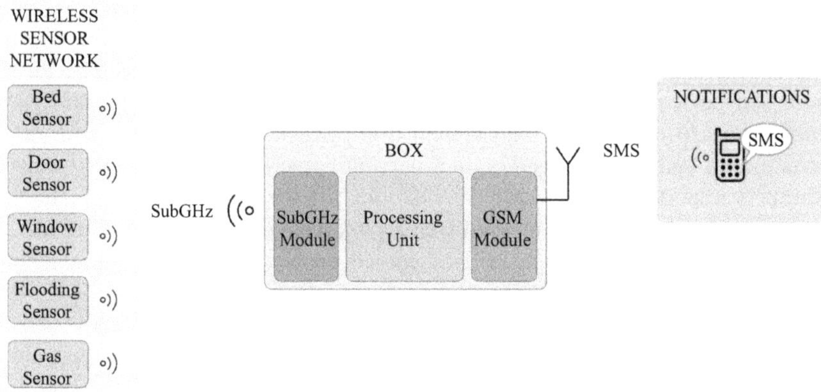

Figure 3.1 UpTech system architecture

components included in the kit was guided by the analysis of the problems related to AD patients, such as cognitive impairment and wandering, and the needs of their caregivers [50], adopting a user-centered design.

As shown in Figure 3.1, each technology kit consisted of a central unit for processing and management, that collected the data transmitted using the Sub-GHz technology by a set of sensors located in different positions inside the home, and processed them, according to specific rules. The wireless sensor network comprises: a sensor to detect the presence in bed of the subject; a sensor to detect flooding on the floor; a sensor to detect smoke or gas leaks; magnetic sensors to detect opening/closing of the door or windows. In addition, a courtesy light is present, which turns on automatically when the person gets up from bed during the night. The central unit processes the events detected by the sensors, and in case of alarm (e.g., flooding or detection of entry door opening) sends to the appointed caregivers an SMS which describes the type of event that generated it.

During the trial, the UpTech kits installed by technicians worked 24/7 without requiring any interventions, and without affecting the patients' habits. The wireless sensors may be easily and quickly installed, and this feature is very useful. In fact, the set up of the kit in the environment shall be completed in a short time, to avoid that the patients see the technicians at work in their homes, and get worried or scared about them, due to the effects of their disease. The trial took place in the Marche Region (Italy), it lasted 12 months and involved 450 dyads, i.e., patient and caregiver couple, divided into groups. All the dyads received three visits by the nurses; a group of them kept periodical phone contacts with the social workers, while the monitoring kits were supplied to a group of around 80 dyads.

During the trial, three assessments have been performed using proper questionnaires, distributed by the nurses during the home visits. The questionnaires mainly included: a section oriented to the patient; a section oriented to the caregiver; a section aimed at evaluating the consumption of socio-health resources by the dyads. In addition, an evaluation survey about the technological kit has been carried out. Thanks to the data collected, it has been possible to know in detail the situation of the patients and their caregivers in the Marche Region. The information obtained concerns for example age, gender, capability of executing ADLs and IADLs, possible behaviour disorders of the patients. As for the caregivers, the type of relation with the patient (e.g., son/daughter, spouse), the perception of the social assistance received, the amount of assistance they provide to the patients. A statistical model has been defined for the estimate of the factors correlated to the Caregiver Burden Inventory (CBI), e.g., the level of caregiver burden. From the study, it emerged for example that the CBI growth is related to the amount of hours dedicated to the assistance, to the condition of son/daughter (with respect to other relatives) and to the inability of performing ADLs. Otherwise, the CBI decreases when social assistance is provided, and when the patients show a good physical condition [51].

Finally, the overall opinion on the kit is positive: some problems have been observed, and the participants provided some useful suggestions to improve the system. The feedbacks have been very important for the design of the new kit employed in the "Tech Home" project, described in Section 3.4.2.2. As concerns the ATs, the trial helped to test the effectiveness and contribution of the developed technology to improve the quality of life of both PwD and their caregivers.

3.4.2.2 Tech Home

The Tech Home system represents an evolution of UpTech, carried out on the basis of the feedbacks obtained from the first project trial.

The system architecture is described in Figure 3.2: the core of the system is the so-called *box*, composed by a processing unit, a sub-GHz module and a GSM-GPRS module. The former module allows the communication with the wireless sensor network, while the latter is used to send notifications and receive configuration messages (SMS). In addition to the original sensors of the UpTech kit, the new version includes other devices: a presence sensor to detect the patient's presence in the bathroom; a magnetic sensor on the refrigerator door to obtain information about eating; temperature and humidity sensors to collect contextual information. The set of sensors detects events and sends them to the central unit, by the sub-GHz communication. At the central unit, data are processed, and if an alarming event has occurred, a notification is sent to the caregiver. The situations considered as alarms are the following ones:

- the door or window is open;
- the patient wakes up and does not get back to bed within a certain time interval (during nighttime);
- the refrigerator door has not been opened for a long time (over a fixed time interval);
- the patient has not accessed a certain area of the house for a defined time interval;
- alarms caused by smoke and water detectors;
- the temperature goes above or below a threshold;
- the humidity rate exceeds a certain threshold.

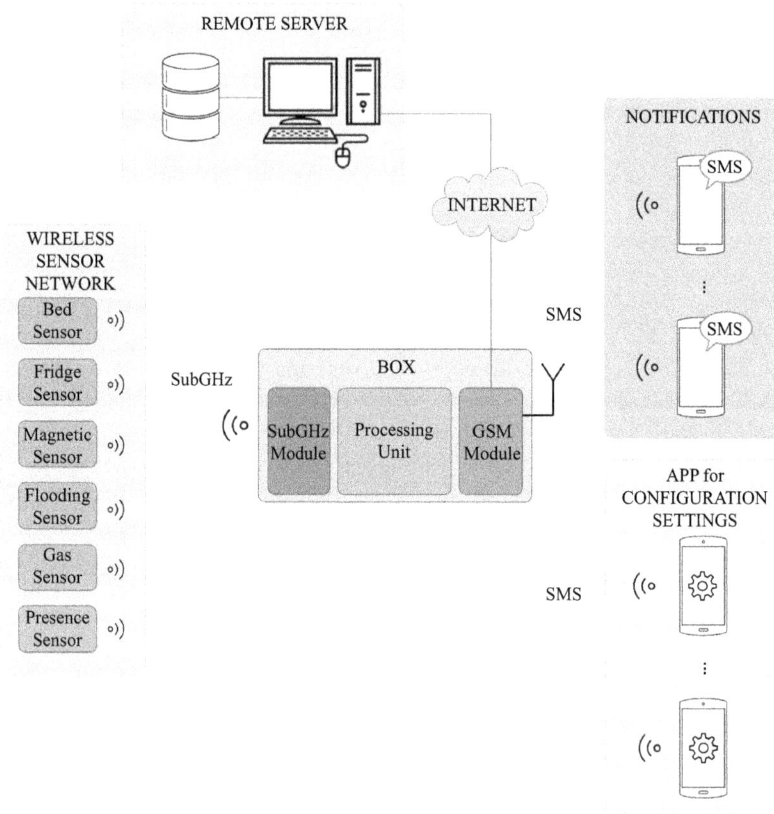

Figure 3.2 Tech Home system architecture

The system foresees the configuration of a list of caregivers' phone numbers: if an alarm is detected, a phone call is performed toward the first number in the caregivers' list, using pre-recorded voice messages. In case of no answer, the box tries to contact the following number, till the end of the list. If none of the contact persons answers, an SMS is sent. Contrary to the alarm management of the UpTech system, in this case a feedback from the caregiver is expected, in order to increase the reliability of the alarm notification delivery. All the events occurred within a 24 h time range are written in a report file, that is sent by the box to the remote server, over the GPRS connection.

The box configuration can be performed by means of a dedicated smartphone application (Figure 3.3). It enables, for example, to save a list of caregivers to be called in case of alarm, to set time intervals and thresholds, to enable/disable sensors notifications and to define some technical parameters. Once the caregiver or installer has set the parameters, they are formatted following a defined protocol and sent to the box via SMS. All the requests performed through the mobile app are written in the daily report generated by the box.

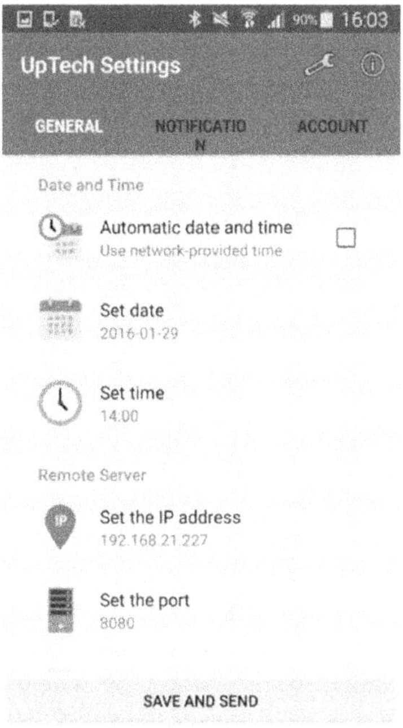

Figure 3.3 Screenshot of the smartphone app for the system configuration (icons provided by Icons8)

At the end of the UpTech project trial, participants filled in an assessment questionnaire that allowed to understand strong and weak aspects of the developed solution, and to implement proper modifications. The main improvements brought are listed below.

- Remote communication toward a server: this feature increases the system reliability, ensuring continuous monitoring, detection of eventual malfunctions and prompt intervention if necessary.
- Mobile app for the dynamic configuration of the system: it makes the configuration easier and user-friendly, and provides more flexibility and adaptation the each user's needs, by allowing on-going modifications.
- Introduction of new sensors to enhance the level of monitoring: a presence sensor monitors the user's presence in a room (for example to verify that he/she enters the bathroom periodically), and a magnetic sensor placed on the refrigerator door can detect its opening, giving information about eating.
- New bed presence and water sensors: the new bed sensor provides a calibration that adapts the sensing to the patient's weight, while the sensor for the flooding detection has been replaced because of false alarms due to high humidity rates.
- Acoustic alarms generated locally have been removed, since they could frighten the users.

- A battery pack for back-up has been added to the box: in case of unexpected energy blackout, the processing unit can continue its normal operation for a certain time interval. Then, if the interruption prolongs over time, it shuts down in a controlled and safe way.
- Reduced box physical dimensions: thanks to a more accurate design, some elements have been removed from the box, that is now less obtrusive than before.

The technological kit has been engineered and the field test phase is ongoing: it is planned to install up to one hundred monitoring kits in the homes of PwD taking part in the trial.

3.4.2.3 UpTech RSA

Unlike the previous solutions, UpTech RSA is designed to monitor the AD patients in nursing homes [52]. Particularly, its purpose is to support the assistance of patients during the night hours, when there is a lack of personnel in the building. Moreover, typically, the night staff is a vulnerable group, receiving less training, supervision and support than day staff, but with a higher level of responsibility [53].

The system architecture is shown in Figure 3.4. As can be seen from the picture, UpTech RSA is characterized by some peculiarities. First of all, in a nursing home, multiple patients are monitored at the same time. For this reason, the system has to manage data coming from several sensor networks. Moreover, different types of sensors are employed, being the physical environment to monitor different from the home one. Specifically, the set of sensors installed in each room enables the following functionalities: door, window and French window opening detection, presence in the bed detection, and presence in the bathroom detection. As in previous cases, the opening of doors and windows is detected through magnetic sensors, the bed presence is recorded using a self-calibrating force sensor, while the presence in the bathroom is detected thanks to a PIR positioned so as to illuminate the whole room.

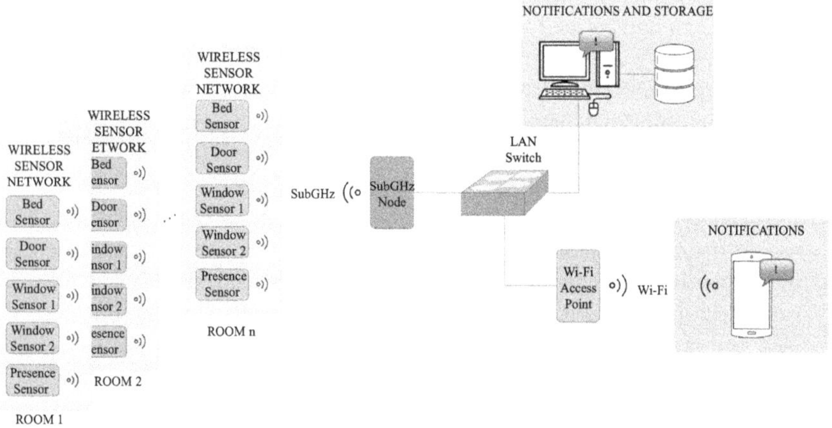

Figure 3.4 UpTech RSA architecture

All these sensors are connected to a gateway through the sub-GHz technology. More specifically, the gateway is a sub-GHz/Ethernet interface and represents the central node that forwards data to a PC located in the nurses' station. Data related to events are saved in a local DB, while those referred to the system operating status are processed and verified in order to ensure the proper functioning of the system.

The notification handling is specifically designed for nurses or health personnel. In fact, two different user interfaces have been used: a desktop interface to monitor patients from the nurses' station, and a mobile application to allow them to receive notifications even when located outside the station, to carry out the caring activities.

At each notification, the smartphone application provides an acoustic alarm and the device vibration, and notifications are structured as a scrollable list of events identified by the name of the sensor, the floor and the room number, as can be seen in Figure 3.5. The corresponding alert level, from low to high, is notified through dots of ascending grey color intensity. Moreover, the sensors or gateway malfunctioning is notified as a gray dot.

UpTech RSA is already available as a prototype. After a first test campaign in the laboratory environment, a second one in the real world followed. The prototype has been installed in a nursing home in Macerata (Italy). Two rooms have been equipped with sensors and monitored for more than three months. In the first room two female patients are housed, only one suffering from AD. The other is a disabled person and cannot move autonomously, thus, just the AD patient's bed is equipped with a force

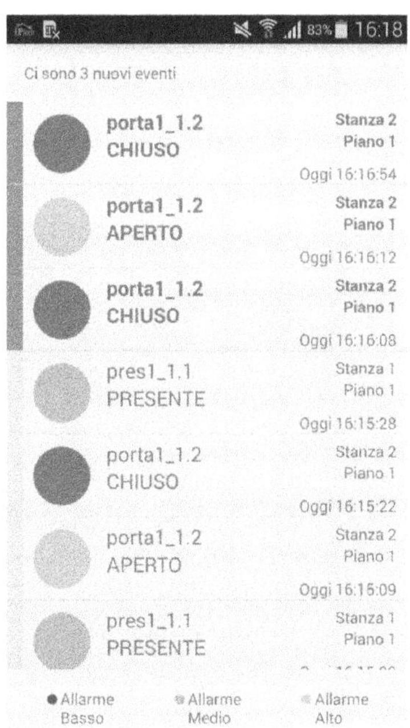

Figure 3.5 Alarm notifications display on the smartphone app

sensor. In the second room a not independent female patient suffering from AD is housed; she moves through a wheelchair. The outcomes of the trial have been positive and the system has proved to be very useful. This is confirmed by answers given by the nurses to an evaluation survey. In fact, some weeks after the installation, 18 nurses were asked about usability and usefulness of the monitoring kit. The 100% of respondents believes the kit is easy to use and recommends it as a monitoring system in nursing homes; 89% of them have an overall positive opinion of it, while only 11% of nurses gives it a medium rating.

The personnel reports that two dangerous episodes occurred during the trial, such as a French window opening and a patient's fall out of the room during the night. In both cases the system has correctly detected and notified the alarming situation, allowing the personnel to react quickly.

In addition to notifying alarm events, the technology described so far is able to store the data acquired by the sensors. Such data can be very useful because they permit to obtain information about the patient's habits and, consequently, to identify any changes or abnormal behaviors.

As an example, in Figure 3.6 a graph of the sleep activity is displayed for the patient in the single room. The sleep activity has been detected considering the activations/deactivations of the bed sensor. The chart shows on the ordinate the days of participation in the trial, while on the abscissa the time expressed as minutes in a day. The sleep activity is represented in a light color. Usually, the patient goes to sleep and wakes up at the same hour, respectively, 06:00 AM–07:00 AM (360–420 min) and 07:00 PM–08:00 PM (1,140–1,200 min). Missing nights in the central part of the graph are due to technical malfunctions of the monitoring system, which have been detected and notified to the personnel, and promptly resolved. Future developments foresee

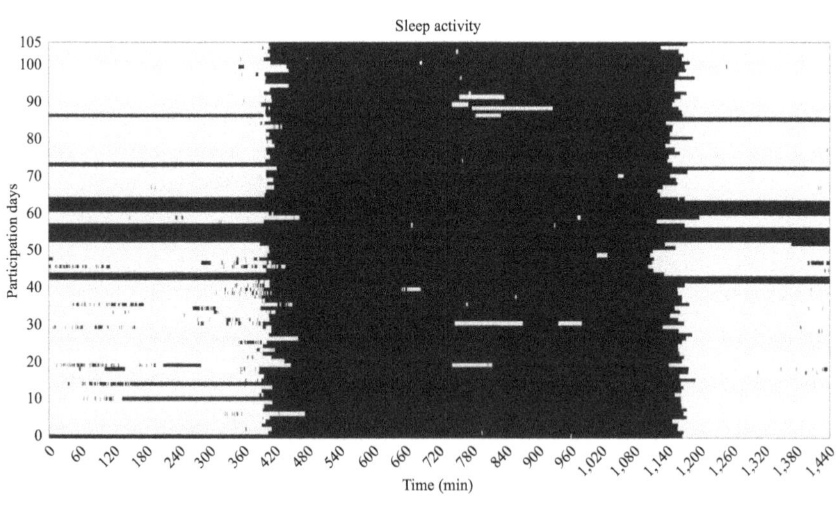

Figure 3.6 Sleep activity representation for the patient in the single room

the implementation of machine learning algorithms for the detection of outliers and anomalies with respect to the patient's usual behaviour.

3.5 Conclusions

The design of assistive technologies for people with needs, a field that began some decades ago and more recently addressed also people with dementia, exhibits slow but steady progress, that led from non-intelligent and primarily single-functional devices, to much more advanced solutions, able to integrate sensing, context-aware automatic reasoning and communication capabilities. However, much still remains to be done, especially because the ultimate success of assistive technology must be measured not only by functional improvement within limited specific domains, but in the perspective of personally meaningful impact on the user's global quality of life. The User Centered Design is a promising direction towards this aim. Although this approach requires greater initial research investment, it ultimately reduces product development time and cost, while simultaneously improving user acceptance and satisfaction. Such an approach deserves urgent research and development priority, to finally obtain a detailed description of both the product design process and the proactive involvement of users with dementia, their families and professional caregivers. In fact, interventions that showed to be effective share some common features: family caregivers are actively involved in the intervention in contrast to passively receiving information; the intervention is tailored and flexible to meet the changing needs of family caregivers during the course of a relative dementia; and the intervention meets the needs not only of caregivers, but of care recipients as well.

More work is needed to ensure that interventions for dementia caregivers are available and accessible to those who need them. Because caregivers and the settings in which they provide care are diverse, more studies are required to define which interventions are most effective for specific situations. Improved tools to personalize services for caregivers, to maximize their benefits, is an emerging area of research. More studies are also needed to explore the effectiveness of interventions in different racial, ethnic and socioeconomic groups, and in different geographical settings.

The above mentioned activities will also contribute to solve another critical issue that needs to be tackled, i.e., the collection of evidence-based clinical and cost-effectiveness data, that will be critical to reimbursement by third-party entities (like public welfare agencies), if widespread acceptance and use of technological resources for alleviating the burden of dementia caring is to become a reality.

References

[1] American Psychiatric Association, "Diagnostic and statistical manual of mental disorders (5th edition)," 2013.

[2] L. E. Hebert, J. Weuve, P. A. Scherr, and D. A. Evans, "Alzheimer disease in the united states (2010–2050) estimated using the 2010 census," *Neurology*, vol. 80, no. 19, pp. 1778–1783, 2013.

[3] Alzheimer's Association, "Early-onset dementia: A national challenge, a future crisis," Report, June 2006. Available at: https://www.alz.org/national/documents/report_earlyonset_full.pdf. [Online; accessed 2 April 2017].

[4] A. D. International, *World Alzheimer Report 2015: The Global Impact of Dementia. An Analysis of Prevalence, Incidence, Cost and Trends*, August ed., London, 2015, from https://www.alz.co.uk/research/WorldAlzheimerReport2015.pdf [Online; accessed 25/01/2017].

[5] S. Carretero, J. Garcès, F. Ródenas, and V. Sanjosé, "The informal caregiver's burden of dependent people: theory and empirical review," *Archives of Gerontology and Geriatrics*, vol. 49, no. 1, pp. 74–79, 2009.

[6] K. Ornstein and J. E. Gaugler, "The problem with 'problem behaviors': a systematic review of the association between individual patient behavioral and psychological symptoms and caregiver depression and burden within the dementia patient–caregiver dyad," *International Psychogeriatrics*, vol. 24, pp. 1536–1552, Oct. 2012.

[7] K. M. Godwin, W. L. Mills, J. A. Anderson, and M. E. Kunik, "Technology-driven interventions for caregivers of persons with dementia: a systematic review," *American Journal of Alzheimer's Disease and Other Dementias*, vol. 28, no. 3, pp. 216–222, 2013.

[8] C. Chiatti, F. Masera, J. Rimland, *et al.*, "The up-tech project, an intervention to support caregivers of Alzheimer's disease patients in Italy: study protocol for a randomized controlled trial," *Trials*, vol. 14, no. 1, 2013.

[9] F. Lattanzio, A. M. Abbatecola, R. Bevilacqua, *et al.* "Advanced technology care innovation for older people in Italy: necessity and opportunity to promote health and wellbeing," *Journal of the American Medical Directors Association*, vol. 15, no. 7, pp. 457–466, 2014.

[10] R. Bevilacqua, E. Felici, F. Marcellini, *et al.*, *Robot-Era Project: Preliminary Results on the System Usability*. Cham: Springer International Publishing, 2015, pp. 553–561.

[11] P. Maresova and B. Klimova, "Supporting technologies for old people with dementia: a review," *IFAC-PapersOnLine*, vol. 48, no. 4, pp. 129–134, 2015.

[12] M. C. Carrillo, E. Dishman, and T. Plowman, "Everyday technologies for Alzheimer's disease care: research findings, directions, and challenges," *Alzheimer's & Dementia*, vol. 5, no. 6, pp. 479–488, Nov. 2009.

[13] T. Patterson, I. Cleland, P. J. Hartin, *et al.*, "Home-based self-management of dementia: closing the loop," in *Inclusive Smart Cities and e-Health*. Berlin: Springer International Publishing, 2015, pp. 232–243.

[14] C. Peterson, N. Prasad, and R. Prasad, "The future of assistive technologies for dementia," *Gerontechnology*, vol. 11, no. 2, p. 259, Jun. 2012.

[15] T. Sugihara, T. Fujinami, R. Phaal, and Y. Ikawa, "Gaps between assistive technologies and dementia care," in *2012 Proceedings of PICMET'12: Technology Management for Emerging Technologies*, Jul. 2012, pp. 3067–3072.

[16] A. DeSantis, A. DelCampo, E. Gambi, *et al.*, "Unobtrusive monitoring of physical activity in AAL – a simple wearable device designed for older adults," in

Proceedings of the First International Conference on Information and Communication Technologies for Ageing Well and e-Health, Lisbon, Portugal, 2015, pp. 200–205.

[17] A. Papetti, M. Iualé, S. Ceccacci, R. Bevilacqua, M. Germani, and M. Mengoni, *Smart Objects: An Evaluation of the Present State Based on User Needs*. Cham: Springer International Publishing, 2014, pp. 359–368.

[18] S. Spinsante, E. Cippitelli, A. DeSantis, *et al.*, *Multimodal Interaction in a Elderly-Friendly Smart Home: A Case Study*. Cham: Springer International Publishing, 2015, pp. 373–386.

[19] N. Beauchamp, A. B. Irvine, J. Seeley, and B. Johnson, "Worksite-based internet multimedia program for family caregivers of persons with dementia," *The Gerontologist*, vol. 45, no. 6, pp. 793–801, 2005.

[20] TeleAlarm, "Telealarm security and telecare," 2016, [Online; accessed 25/01/2017]. [Online]. Available: http://www.telealarm.com/en.

[21] Tunstall, "Tunstall healthcare," 2016, [Online; accessed 25/01/2017]. [Online]. Available: http://www.tunstall.co.uk/.

[22] "Careinnovations," 2016, [Online; accessed 25/01/2017]. [Online]. Available: http://www.careinnovations.com/qtug/.

[23] "iSens (Projectname INAT)," 2016, [Online; accessed 25/01/2017]. [Online]. Available: https://www.hslu.ch/en/lucerne-school-of-engineering-architecture/research/kompetenzzentren/ihomelab/projekte/.

[24] S. Pal and C. Abhayaratne, "Video-based activity level recognition for assisted living using motion features," in *Proceedings of the Ninth International Conference on Distributed Smart Cameras*, ser. ICDSC'15. New York, NY: ACM, 2015, pp. 62–67.

[25] Y. Li, K. C. Ho, and M. Popescu, "A microphone array system for automatic fall detection," *IEEE Transactions on Biomedical Engineering*, vol. 59, no. 5, pp. 1291–1301, May 2012.

[26] S. Gasparrini, E. Cippitelli, S. Spinsante, and E. Gambi, "A depth-based fall detection system using a Kinect® sensor," *Sensors*, vol. 14, no. 2, pp. 2756–2775, 2014.

[27] S. A. Bridenbaugh and R. W. Kressig, "Laboratory review: the role of gait analysis in seniors' mobility and fall prevention," *Gerontology*, vol. 57, no. 3, pp. 256–264, 2011.

[28] ekahau, "ekahau wi-fi rtls, active rfid tracking solutions and wi-fi site survey, wlan planning tools," 2016, [Online; accessed 25/01/2017]. [Online]. Available: http://www.ekahau.com/.

[29] iBeaconInsider, "Your guide to ibeacon technology," 2016, [Online; accessed 25/01/2017]. [Online]. Available: http://www.ibeacon.com/.

[30] iWearGPS, "iweargps, sos technology," 2016, [Online; accessed 25/01/2017]. [Online]. Available: http://iweargps.com/.

[31] NEAT, "Nemo portable alarm trigger with gps and gsm," 2016, [Online; accessed 25/01/2017]. [Online]. Available: http://www.neat-group.com/se/en/carephones/nemo/.

[32] Lively, "Emergency medical alert system," 2016, [Online; accessed 25/01/2017]. [Online]. Available: http://www.mylively.com/.
[33] sen.se, "mother. whatever you need, whenever you want," 2016, [Online; accessed 25/01/2017]. [Online]. Available: https://sen.se/mother/.
[34] Careinnovations, "Smart sensor technology that measures and interprets patients' activities of daily living (adls)," 2016, [Online; accessed 25/01/2017]. [Online]. Available: http://www.careinnovations.com/quietcare/.
[35] "Technology for Aging in Place 2016 – Market Overview," https://www.ageinplacetech.com/files/aip/MarketOverview20Feb-2016-Final_1.pdf, 2016, [Online; accessed 25/01/2017].
[36] C. Schneider, V. Willner, M. Feichtenschlager, A. Andrushevich, and L. Spiru, "Collecting user requirements for electronic assistance for people with dementia: a case study in three countries," in *2013 Proceedings of the eHealth Conference*, Vienna, Austria, May 2013, pp. 1–6.
[37] I. Asghar, S. Cang, and H. Yu, "A systematic mapping study on assitive technologies for people with dementia," in *2015 Ninth International Conference on Software, Knowledge, Information Management and Applications (SKIMA)*, Kathmandu, Nepal, Dec. 2015, pp. 1–8.
[38] Alzheimer's Society, "Assistive technology – devices to help with everyday living," 2016, [Online; accessed 25/01/2017]. [Online]. Available: https://www.alzheimers.org.uk/site/scripts/documents_info.php?documentID=109.
[39] G. Tegart, E. Harvey, A. Livingstone, C. Martin, E. Ozanne, and J. Soar, "Assistive Health Technologies for Independent Living," Report for the Australian Council of Learned Academies, Tech. Rep., 2014.
[40] D. Silver, M. Winchcombe, and H. Pinnock, "Towards a successful consumer market for electronic assisted living technologies (eALT)," Research findings from the COMODAL project, Tech. Rep., 2014.
[41] G. Ward and S. Ray, "Unlocking the potential of the younger older consumer: consumer preferences and the assisted living market," Research findings from the COMODAL project, Tech. Rep., 2014.
[42] D. F. Mahoney, B. J. Tarlow, and R. N. Jones, "Effects of an automated telephone support system on caregiver burden and anxiety: findings from the reach for tlc intervention study," *The Gerontologist*, vol. 43, no. 4, pp. 556–567, 2003.
[43] R. Bevilacqua, M. Di Rosa, E. Felici, V. Stara, F. Barbabella, and L. Rossi, *Towards an Impact Assessment Framework for ICT-Based Systems Supporting Older People: Making Evaluation Comprehensive Through Appropriate Concepts and Metrics*. Cham: Springer International Publishing, 2014, pp. 215–222.
[44] M. P. Cutchin, "The process of mediated aging-in-place: a theoretically and empirically based model," *Social Science & Medicine*, vol. 57, no. 6, pp. 1077–1090, Sep. 2003.
[45] M. Amiribesheli and A. Bouchachia, "Smart homes design for people with dementia," in *2015 International Conference on Intelligent Environments*. Institute of Electrical & Electronics Engineers (IEEE), Jul. 2015.

[46] D. Li, H. W. Park, M. Piao, and K. H. Ryu, "The design and partial implementation of the dementia-aid monitoring system based on sensor network and cloud computing platform," in *Applied Computing & Information Technology*. Springer International Publishing, Dec. 2015, pp. 85–100.

[47] W. Bourennane, Y. Charlon, F. Bettahar, E. Campo, and D. Esteve, "Homecare monitoring system: a technical proposal for the safety of the elderly experimented in an Alzheimer's care unit," *IRBM*, vol. 34, no. 2, pp. 92–100, Apr. 2013.

[48] H. Aloulou, M. Mokhtari, T. Tiberghien, *et al.*, "Deployment of assistive living technology in a nursing home environment: methods and lessons learned," *BMC Medical Informatics and Decision Making*, vol. 13, no. 1, p. 42, 2013.

[49] D. M. Taub, S. B. Leeb, E. C. Lupton, R. T. Hinman, J. Zeisel, and S. Blackler, "The escort system: a safety monitor for people living with Alzheimer's disease," *IEEE Pervasive Computing*, vol. 10, no. 2, pp. 68–77, Apr. 2011.

[50] F. Barbabella, C. Chiatti, F. Masera, *et al.*, "Experimentation of an integrated system of services and aal solutions for Alzheimer's disease patients and their caregivers in the Marche region: the up-tech project (in Italian)," 2013, Italian Conference on Ambient Assisted Living (ForItAAL).

[51] U. R. Team, "Sperimentazione di un sistema integrato di servizi nell'ambito della continuita' assistenziale a soggetti affetti da Alzheimer e loro familiari," Report finale del progetto di ricerca Uptech, Tech. Rep., 2014.

[52] L. Montanini, L. Raffaeli, A. DeSantis, *et al.*, "Overnight supervision of Alzheimer's disease patients in nursing homes – system development and field trial," in *Proceedings of the International Conference on Information and Communication Technologies for Ageing Well and e-Health*, 2016, pp. 15–25.

[53] D. Kerr, C. Cunningham, and H. Wilkinson, *Supporting Older People in Care Homes at Night*. Joseph Rowntree Foundation, York, UK, 2008.

Chapter 4

Wearable sensors for gesture analysis in smart healthcare applications

Abdul Haleem Butt, Alessandra Moschetti*, Laura Fiorini, Paolo Dario, and Filippo Cavallo*

Abstract

Technological solutions represent new opportunities to help elderly people and their caregivers in daily life. Understanding human behavior becomes thus essential in Ambient Assisted Living field especially for prevention and monitoring applications. In particular, recognition of human gestures is important to deliver personalized service to keep elderly people independent, while being monitored by caregivers. This chapter aims to underline the importance of recognizing behavior and in particular gesture in order to monitor older persons. An overview of the gesture recognition applications in AAL is therefore presented with a focus on the existing technologies used to capture hand gestures. Algorithms for data processing and classification are also described. Finally, an example of daily gesture recognition in AAL is presented where different gestures are recognized by mean of SensHand.

4.1 Introduction: healthcare and technology

The population of the EU is expected to reach 526 million by 2050, and the demographic old-age dependency ratio (number of people age 65 or above compared to those age 15–64) projected to rise from the current 28% to 50% by 2060 [1]. This evident demographic shift foretells that understanding healthy aging and age-related diseases will be a future challenge. Additionally, the decrease of working-age population will lead to an increase in the demand for nurse practitioners (+94% in 2025) [2] and physician's assistants (+72% in 2025) [3], as well as an increased need for a higher level of care and for future assistance. Today, having a good quality of care and highly sustainable health-care services are increasingly imperative in EU countries [4].

*Both the authors contributed equally.

Several research efforts conducted in recent years highlight the primary needs of elderly people and stakeholders [5,6]. Elderly citizens suffer from cognitive and physical disorders due to natural decline, and mental and physical impairments [6]. People with cognitive disorders could have problems in keeping control of their lives, and in effect, recent studies correlate changes in the daily behavior of older persons with cognitive problems [7]. Additionally, older individuals need to reduce the risk of accidents at home and may require assistance in managing chronic diseases [5]. Due to all these reasons, over the past few years, requests for home-care services have increased [8].

The main objective of Ambient Assisted Living (AAL) is to provide adequate technological solutions which could increase the level of quality of life [9]. AAL applications span both helping the different stakeholders in preventing accidents and monitoring elderly people at home [10]. Recent advances in mobile Internet, the Internet of Things (IoT), and telehealth services increase the perception abilities of the devices, thus providing an efficient "Continuum of Care" and assistance everywhere. The users will be monitored constantly, without the necessity for a person to live with them [11]. In effect, a recent study [12] underlines that the improvement in the management of health conditions, remote feedback from nurses, and feeling of safety and self-confidence about their status are all improving the use and acceptance of telehealth technologies.

The understanding of human movements, behavior, and body language is of obvious importance in AAL applications. It can assist in using technological solutions for prevention or monitoring and can also help the communication between the users and the technological devices.

This chapter presents a general overview of the importance of the recognition of human gestures to deliver personalized and efficient services to promote the independent living of elderly individuals. After a brief introduction about smart sensors (Section 4.2) and gesture recognition applications in AAL (Section 4.3), the authors describe the primary technologies used to capture the hand motion (Section 4.4), data processing, and classification algorithms used in gesture recognition (Section 4.5). Additionally, the authors present a concrete application of gesture recognition in AAL field (Section 4.6). Finally, Section 4.7 concludes the work.

4.2 Growth of smart sensors, wearables, and IoT

The rising demand for sustainable healthcare systems has increased the importance of AAL developments, services, and products. The market for medical electronics is expected to reach USD 4.41 billion by 2022 [13], whereas the smart home market, which has been experiencing steady growth, is expected to reach USD 121.73 billion by 2022 [14].

Similarly, the telehealth market was valued at $2.2 billion in 2015 and is predicted to reach $6.5 billion by 2020, with an annual growth rate of 24.2% [15]. The home healthcare industry is also testing tele-homecare and tele-monitoring services that represent a valuable opportunity to balance quality of care with cost control. In effect, according to [12], the possibility to be monitored continuously and the evidence of reduced costs are considered some of the facilitators of telehealth. In this manner, caregivers and family could be connected constantly by smartphone, tablet, or other connected device.

According to [16], more than 10,000 healthcare apps are available in the Apple/Google store. These statistics also reveals that approximately 85% of doctors use smartphones and medical apps, and 80% of them would like their patients to monitor their health status at home. Moreover, the digital impact on user experience is clear, as more than 78% of users are interested in mobile-health solutions.

The number of worldwide mobile subscriptions was equal to 7.3 billion in 2015 and is predicted to reach 9 billion in 2021 with an annual growth rate of 5%. We are now living in the IoT era, where not only are people connected to Internet, but also the number of connected devices was equal to 15 billion in 2015 and is expected to reach 28 billion in 2021 with an annual growth rate of 27% [17].

Wearable devices are now coming to market with form factors that increase comfort during various daily activities. CCS Insight has updated its outlook on the future of wearable tech, indicating that it expects 411 million smart wearable devices to be sold in 2019 and that fitness and activity trackers will account for more than 50% of the unit sales. Particularly, smartwatches will account for almost half of wearables revenue in 2019 [18].

All these smart devices can provide a significant amount of information that could be used in the AAL context to support the understanding of human movements, behavior, and body language, without being invasive, but simply as a part of daily living.

4.3 Application scenarios

Recognition of human movements and gestures plays an important role in AAL solutions. Using them, caregivers and family could monitor and assist elderly persons. In particular, different scenarios can be identified that span from human–robot interaction (HRI) to monitoring applications, as shown in Figure 4.1.

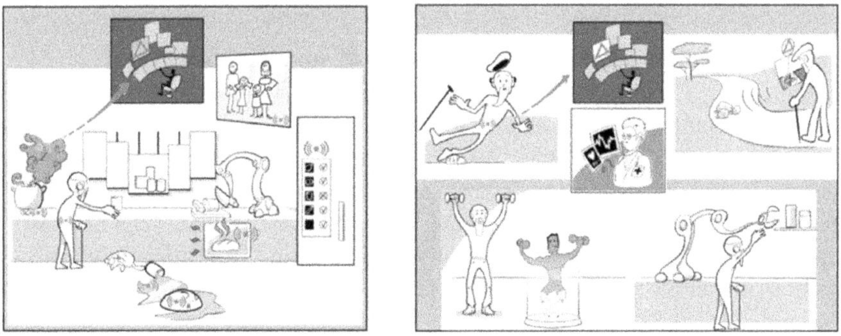

Figure 4.1 Example of AAL scenarios

Prevention of physical and cognitive degeneration

Typical AAL scenarios that involve the use of gesture recognition systems are the ones that aim at preventing early degeneration or dangerous situations by stimulating cognitive and physical abilities [9]. AAL solutions can help elderly people by providing personalized games, made also of different sensors that can detect human movements. In this way, elderly individuals, and others as well, can perform special games that are enjoyable and also provide assistance with physical and cognitive exercises. Through recognition of human movements, caregivers will be able to determine if the person is doing the movement correctly. In this way, people will be able to perform exercises and activities while being monitored by experts. Thanks to these applications, elderly people will be able to train themselves and keep themselves fit, decreasing the risk of degeneration of physical and cognitive abilities [5].

Gesture recognition in monitoring applications

Recognition of movements and gestures plays an important role in monitoring applications, as well. This recognition can assist both in monitoring daily activities and in rehabilitation purposes. Elderly people living alone can change their habits, and this can be seen as a first symptom of a degeneration in cognitive abilities. Often, people with dementia forget to eat and drink or to carry out simple activities of daily living such as personal hygiene behaviors [7]. Having the ability to recognize daily gestures would allow remote monitoring of elderly people to determine whether people can still maintain their daily routines [19]. Alternatively, many persons, and in particular, the elderly, could have to perform exercises at home as assessment tools or for rehabilitation purposes. In this case, the recognition of movements and gestures could help in enabling a continuum of care. After the first training sessions accomplished with the therapist, the patient could perform the activities at home while being monitored. In this way, the user could increase the amount of sessions spent doing the exercises, without the need for a session with the physician [6].

Gesture recognition to control robots and smart appliances

Gesture recognition could also be used to control smart appliances, thanks to the recognition of different movements [6]. These recognition abilities could be used to interact with robots or other devices to enable the people to work longer or continue engaging in personal hobbies and activities that can become difficult to perform after a certain age. Concerning the work, AAL solutions can be used to compensate for sensory and motor deficits, preventing work-related injuries as well. To maneuver heavy or large objects, a remotely controlled robotic arm could be used, instead of a joystick or mouse, by recognizing the gesture the worker is making [6].

Gesture recognition in human–robot interaction

One of the challenges in HRI is to make the robot understand human behavior as it occurs in human–human interaction. Thus, the robot could be able to perceive the action or intention of the user without the person communicating directly to the robot. Inter-personal communication includes non-verbal cues, such as facial expressions, movements, and hand gestures that are used to express feeling and give feedback. Having the abilities to sense and respond appropriately to the users is important to tailor the content of the interaction, increasing the robot's social abilities [11]. The robot could be able to perceive what the user is doing, whether he is eating or drinking or talking to somebody, or simply alone on the sofa becoming bored; in this way, it could approach the user in a tailored manner and attempt to interact properly.

4.4 Gesture recognition technology

The motion capture of human gestures is quite complex due to independent movements of the five fingers [20]. Thus, the technologies related to the capture of gestures should be developed to be fully reliable and highly sensitive, with a low level of invasiveness to minimize the discomfort of the monitoring task. In recent years, many devices based on cameras and inertial sensors have been created to recognize nonverbal behaviors that are important in human communication [21]. Some of them are research products, and others are available on the market. However, most of the developed systems present strong limitations. For instance, regarding cameras, the system based on the three-dimensional (3-D) infrared camera for finger recognition, or other devices based on camera recognition, suffer from line-of-sight obstructions and have heavy computation requirements [22]. Recent research based on 3-D depth sensors, such as the Leap Motion controller (LMC) and Microsoft Kinetic sensor, demonstrate a high degree of segmentation and 3-D hand gesture recognition [23].

In contrast, wearable sensors overcome the limitation of obstruction and light. Being worn by the user, they receive information directly from the movement of the user. However, to use this type of sensor, the user has to wear something on the hand, which can be felt as cumbersome and can limit the ability to perform gestures in a natural way [24]. However, thanks to the miniaturization and affordability of these sensors, particularly of Inertial Measurement Units (IMUs), wearable sensors have demonstrated good potential in recognizing activities [25]. The combination of different types of sensors can improve the accuracy of recognition tasks, but in the case of wearable sensors, it is important to always pay attention to obtrusiveness, maintaining a good trade-off between recognition performance and invasiveness [26].

In this section, some technological solutions, also commercially available, are introduced and described to provide a general overview of the current solutions used for hand gesture recognition.

4.4.1 SensHand

The SensHand is a device developed by Cavallo *et al.* [27,28] in 2013. This device is composed of four, nine-axis inertial sensor units to be worn on the hand as rings and bracelet. In particular, three modules are designed to be worn on three fingers (typically thumb, index, and middle finger), and one module is designed to be worn on the wrist.

The SensHand has gone through different improvements over the years (see Figure 4.2). The last version is made of four inertial sensors integrated into four INEMO-M1 boards with dedicated STM32F103xE family microcontrollers (ARM 32-bit Cortex™-M3 CPU, from STMicroelectronics, Milan, Italy). Each module includes a LSM303DLHC (six-axis geomagnetic module, dynamically user-selectable full scale acceleration, and a magnetic field, from STMicroelectronics, Milan, Italy), an L3G4200D (three-axis digital gyroscope, user-selectable angular rate, from STMicroelectronics, Milan, Italy), and I2C digital output. The integration of these sensors enables 3-D mapping of the motion.

A Controller Area Network standard is used to implement module coordination and data synchronization. The module placed on the wrist is the coordinator of the system: it collects data and transmits them through the Bluetooth V3.0 communication protocol via the SPBT2632C1A (STMicroelectronics, Milan, Italy) Class 1 module toward a generic control station. A small, rechargeable, and light Li-Ion battery supplies power to the device. This battery is integrated in the coordinator module. A fourth-order low-pass digital filter with a cutoff frequency of 5 Hz has been implemented and can be used to remove high-frequency noise and tremor frequency bands in real time [29]. Data are collected on a PC by means of a custom interface developed in C# language. This interface, beyond collecting the data, allows selection of a low-pass filter if desired and the acquisition frequency. Data can be sent at 100 Hz or 50 Hz, depending on the application.

The interface, together with embedded firmware, allows calibration of the three sensors by following some simple rules indicated by the interface (that follows the indication given by the manufacturer of the sensors). In this way, it is possible to calibrate the sensors easily, without reprogramming the device, and removing offsets and sensitivity that can affect the measurements.

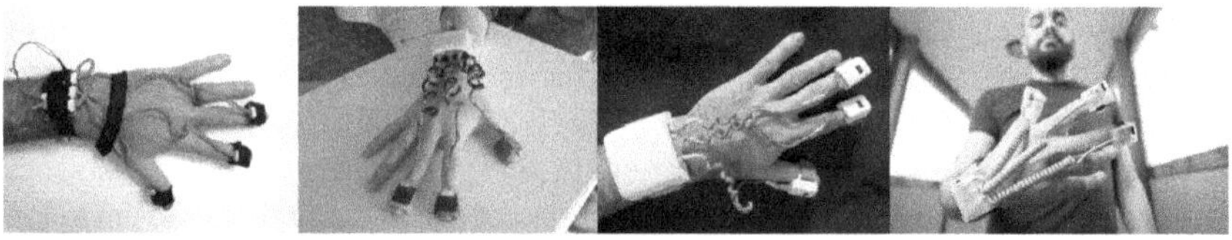

Figure 4.2 Different version of the SensHand

4.4.2 Other gloves

Over the past 30 years or more, researchers have begun developing wearable devices, particularly glove-based systems, to recognize hand gestures. Different working principles have been studied during these years to find a good trade-off between precision, accuracy, and obtrusiveness [30].

Glove-based system

Much attention has been given to glove-based systems because of the natural fit of developing something to be worn on the hand to measure hand movement and finger bending. A glove-based system can be defined as: "a system composed of an array of sensors, electronics for data acquisition/processing and power supply, and a support for the sensors that can be worn on the user's hand" [30]. The various devices can differ based on sensor technologies (i.e. piezoresistive, fiber optic, Hall effect, etc.), number of sensors per finger, sensor support (i.e. cloth or mechanical support), sensor location (i.e. hand joints, fingertip positions, etc.), and others [30]. A typical example of a glove-based system is the CyberGlobe, a cloth device with 18 or 22 piezo-resistive sensors that measures the flexion and the abduction/adduction of the hand joints (depending on the number of sensors, the measurable movements increase). It is considered one of the most accurate commercial systems [30] and has provided good results in recognizing sign language based on the biomechanical characteristics of the movement of the hand [31,32]. CyberGlove showed good results also in applications of robot control and 3-D modelling [33].

Another example of a glove-based system is the 5DT Glove, which is based on optical fiber flexor sensors. The bending of the fingers is measured by measuring the intensity of the returned light indirectly [30]. Each finger has a sensor that measures the overall flexion of the finger. This device is famous for application in virtual reality [33,34].

Other examples of glove-based systems used for sign language include cloth-supported bend sensors based on the Hall Effect mounted together with an accelerometer [35] as well as flex and contact sensors [36]. Carbonaro *et al.* [37] added textile electrodes and an inertial motion unit to the deformation sensors of the glove-based device to add emotion recognition made through electrodermal activity.

IMU-based system

Even though glove-based systems can be very accurate in measuring hand degrees of freedom, they can also be perceived as cumbersome by users because they reduce the dexterity and natural movements. To reduce the invasiveness of the wearable sensors, different technologies have been introduced to recognize hand and finger gestures. One of the proposed solutions introduced the use of IMUs to recognize gestures. In particular, these sensors are worn on the hand to perceive the movements made by the fingers and the hand. The SensHand technology previously described belongs to this category of sensor. Moreover, Bui *et al.* [38] used the AcceleGlove with an added sensor on the back of the hand to recognize postures in Vietnamese Sign Language. In this way, they were able to evaluate the angle between the fingers and the palm and use it for identifying the gesture made.

Kim *et al.* [39] developed a device composed of three three-axis accelerometers, worn on two fingers and on the back of the hand to recognize gestures. With the help of these sensors, they reconstructed the kinematic chain of the hand, allowing the device to recognize simple gestures. In addition, an accelerometer and a gyroscope were used on the back of the hand by Amma *et al.* [40] to recognize 3-D-space handwriting gestures.

Lei *et al.* [41] implemented a wearable ring with an accelerometer to recognize 12 one-stroke finger gestures, extracting temporal and frequency features. The chosen gestures were used to control different appliances in the house [42].

Wearing two three-axis accelerometers on the thumb and on the index finger, Hsieh *et al.* [43] were able to recognize some simple gestures made using these fingers. Using a nine-axis inertial measurement unit, Roshandel *et al.* [44] were able to recognize nine different gestures with four different classifiers.

EMG-based and hybrid systems

New sensors have been developed to read the surface electromyography (sEMG), which is the recording of the muscle activity from the surface, detectable by surface electrodes. In recent years, attention has been paid to this kind of signal to recognize hand and finger gestures. Various technical aspects have been investigated to determine the optimal placement of the electrodes, and select the optimal features for the more appropriate classifier [45]. Naik *et al.* [45] used sEMG to recognize the flection of the fingers, both alone and combined, obtaining good results (accuracy <0.84). Using the same signal, Jung *et al.* [46] developed a new device that uses air pressure sensors and air bladders to measure the EMG signal.

To increase the number and the kind of gestures to be recognized, often different sensors are combined together. Frequently, EMG is combined with inertial sensors worn on the forearm to increase the amount of information obtained by the device. Wolf *et al.* [47] presented the BioSleeve, a device made of sEMG sensors and an IMU to be worn on the forearm. By coupling these two types of sensor, the authors were able to recognize 16 hand gestures, corresponding to various finger and wrist positions that were then used to command robotic platforms. Lu *et al.* [48] uses a similar combination of sensors to recognize 19 predefined gestures to control a mobile phone, achieving average accuracy of 0.95 in user-dependent testing. Georgie *et al.* [49] fused the signals of an IMU worn on the wrist with EMG at the forearm to recognize a total of 12 hand and finger gestures with a recognition rate of 0.743.

4.4.3 Leap motion

The Leap Motion Controller (LMC) is a commercially available optical device that can detect the hand motion and position in the 3-D space. Its weight is 45 g and it is composed of three light emitting diodes (LEDs) and two infrared (IR) cameras with depth sensing abilities (resolution of 640×240 each). Both IR cameras are a distance of 20 mm from the center of the LMC, as depicted in Figure 4.3(a). The field of view in the hemispherical area is approximately 150°.

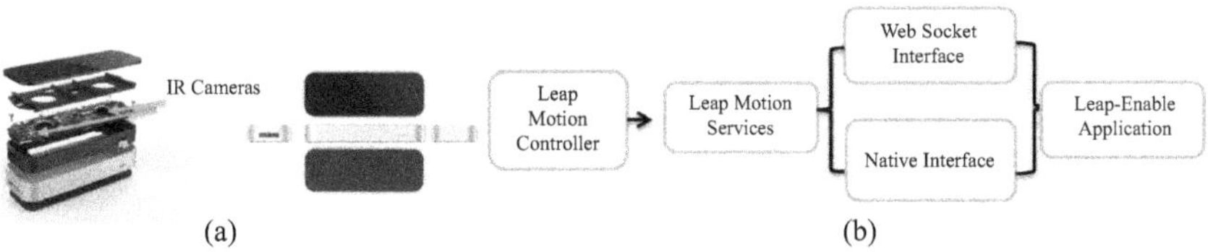

Figure 4.3 (a) Internal structure of leap motion controller and (b) leap motion controller system architecture

The information regarding the user's hand, fingers, and gestures is captured as long as the hand is between 25 mm and 600 mm above the center of the sensor. The hand position captured is relative to the center of LMC [50].

The Leap Motion software development kit (SDK) allows access of the data for hand direction, speed, and rotation, in time-dependent frames with the average frequency of 100 Hz/s, which is considered adequate to capture the movement of the human hand with a high degree of accuracy. For hand movement detection, LMC software uses an internal model of the human hand to estimate the position of the hand, fingers, and gestures, even if the hand is not visible. This model uses dedicated algorithms to collect the information from the visible part of the hand and past observations to calculate the most likely position [51]. LMC also is able to detect the motion of each finger through dedicated algorithms. This aspect represents one of the most important advantages of LMC, which make it more convenient for the different applications.

Leap motion provides two types of APIs to acquire the data from LMC: native interface and WebSocket interface (Figure 4.3(b)). The native interface provides dynamic loaded libraries (DLL). These libraries contain sets of classes and datastructure which allows collection and analysis of data from the device. These libraries can be connected directly with C++ and Objective-C applications, or through one of the language bindings provided for Java, C#, and Python [51].

The WebSocket interface allows the interaction with LMC through the web server and web browser. The communication protocol is hypertext transfer protocol (HTTP), and the messages are codified in JavaScript object notation messages (JSON) to be easy for humans to read and write [51].

4.4.4 Smartwatch

Smartwatches are commercial, wearable devices capable of measuring physiological parameters like heart rate variability and temperature and capable of estimating the movement of the wrist by means of three-axial accelerometers. These devices allow a continual monitoring of the user's daily activities. The acquired information could be analyzed and used for different purposes such as wellness, safety, gesture recognition, and the detection of an activity/inactivity period [52]. Today, many different smartwatches are available on the market. Apple watch, Samsung Gear S3, Huawei Watch, and Polar M600 are several examples.

Because of the smartwatch's sensor functionality, the device enables new and innovative applications that expand the original application field. Since 2001 [53], researchers have been paying attention to the movement of the wrist to estimate hand gestures. Now, smartwatches are offering a concrete possibility to exploit the recognition of gestures in real applications. For instance, Wile *et al.* [54] use smartwatches to identify and monitor the Parkinson Disease's postural tremor in 41 subjects. The results suggest that the smartwatch could measure the tremor with good correlation with respect to other devices. In other research, Liu *et al.* [55] fuse the information of an inertial sensor placed on the wrist with a Kinect camera to identify different gestures (agree, question mark, shake hand) to improve the interaction with a companion robot. Ahanathapillai *et al.* [56] use an Android smartwatch to recognize common daily activities such as walking and ascending/descending stairs. The parameters that are extracted in this work include activity level and step count. The achievements confirm good recognition of all the selected features.

4.5 Description of the main approaches for gesture classification

The data collected from the devices should be properly processed to extract significant features and then used to build a recognition model via machine learning techniques. This section describes the main features which could be extracted from lip motion devices and IMU glove (SensHand), and discusses the main techniques to select and classify the features adopted in AAL applications.

4.5.1 Features used in gesture recognition for AAL

To use the signals coming from the different devices, it is necessary to extract significant features, which means: "filtering relevant information and obtaining quantitative measures that allow signals to be compared" [25].

Several features could be extracted from data, depending on the technology used. In general, a statistical and a structural approach have been proposed to extract features from the time series. The former approach uses quantitative characteristics of the data (e.g. Fourier Transform) while the latter uses interrelationships among the data. Whether to use one or the other depends on the signal to be analyzed [25]. However, the selection of features depends primarily on the application of the gesture recognition system. In this context, the authors will present concrete applications of various sets of features in different AAL solutions.

As described in the previous section, LMC devices used depth imaging to detect the hand motion by using a hand skeletal model. Furthermore, appropriate depth segmentation techniques, based on a computer vision algorithms, are able to reconstruct hand motion, even if the full hand is not completely visible [57]. By default, LMC provides the time-domain features from captured hand movements and can recognize four different gestures.

The time-domain features include the physical properties of the hand, arm, and fingers; motions like velocity, speed, distance, angle (pitch, roll, yaw), position (x, y, z), length, and width; grab strength (hand opening and closing strength); and pinch strength (colliding strength between fingers).

The recognized gestures are screen tap, key tap, swipe, and circle; they are used to access specific movement patterns. The movement parameters provided by LMC for circle gesture are minimum radius (mm) and minimum arc length (rad). For swipe gesture, the parameters are minimum velocity and minimum length. Finally, for screen tap and key tap, the extracted features are minimum velocity and finger movements.

However, some problems were experienced with the LMC. The device cannot detect the fingertip parameters when two (or more) fingers are very close to each other or the hand is in neutral position. The LMC will stop detecting the hands and fingers if the hands are tilted and the fingers are no longer in the field of view of the device. Additionally, LMC often loses the focus during the hand motion, which makes the features extraction procedures unreliable.

As confirmed from the state of the art, LMC gesture recognition is used in the different rehabilitation games. Exploiting the gamification paradigm [58], it has been introduced in the rehabilitation therapy of stroke patients to motivate them to pull, push, and grasp.

LMC is also often used to estimate the essential tremor in aging people and in patients with Parkinson's disease (PwPD). The traditional clinical assessment is still lacking in automated procedures able to quantify the severity of the hand tremor. In this context, LMC could represent a valid tool which could be used by clinicians. It is able to detect high-frequency movements such as tremor of the fingers and hand. Chen *et al.* [59] showed that the amplitude measured by LMC presents a strong linear correlation with the amplitude revealed by an accelerometer. In [60], LMC was used to overcome the limitations of the Kinetic sensor to assess the small movements of the PwPD hand such as rest tremor and postural tremor.

Lu *et al.* [23] used hand palm direction, fingertip positions, palm center position, and other relevant points to track the dynamic movements of daily activities such as opening and closing the hand, movement of fingers, hand movement in circle, and finger movements in upward or downward direction without requiring extra computation. Moreover, in the same study, other features were extracted from the hand gesture: Poke, Pinch, Pull, Scrape, Slap, Press, Cut, Circle, Key Tap, and Mow.

Of note, IMU-based wearable devices allow extraction of the features in time domain, frequency domain, time–frequency domain, and other based on the specific application [61].

The time-domain features are the general statistical features of a signal. The ones that are often used are mean, standard deviation, variance, mean absolute deviation (MAD), root mean square (RMS), median, zero crossing, interquartile range (IQR), correlation between axis, entropy, and kurtosis [25,62]. These features typically play an essential role in movement classification and detection tasks if most discriminative features are not known.

The frequency domain signal provides frequency patterns of different activities. The frequency domain features analyze the frequency performance of the sensor signals, which is usually the periodicity of the signal over a long duration. Typical frequency domain features are the Fourier Transform, the spectral energy, and the Discrete Cosine Transform [25,62]. Some of these features also can be employed when IMUs are used for activity recognition.

The study of Zhang *et al.* [63] showed the potential of IMU to access the motor disorder of upper limbs in PwPD and stroke patients. Objective assessment of upper limbs for post-stroke patients with the dynamic time wrapping signal from the x, y, z-axes was estimated. The placement of the wireless IMU sensor was on the affected hand wrist. A novel single-index-based assessment approach for quantitative upper-limb mobility evaluation was proposed for post-stroke rehabilitation. Similarly, in 2013 Cavallo *et al.* [27] used the SensHand device to access the PwPD patients' tremors. To evaluate the severity of the disease, different biomechanical parameters were evaluated from the signals coming from the accelerometers and the gyroscopes. In particular, according to the different exercises performed by the patients, the following features were extracted by Rovini *et al.* [64] using the SensHand: movement frequency, movement amplitude, movement velocity, variability of the movement in frequency and amplitude, energy expenditure, signal power, fundamental frequency, and percentage of power band. The results of the preliminary study [65] suggest a strong correlation with some biomechanical features and the clinical scale, thus providing an objective assessment of the disease.

4.5.2 Features selections

Large-scale and high-dimensional data acquired from these wearable sensors required conversion of this data to meaningful information. Typically, these high dimensionalities are associated with high levels of noise. The two main causes of noise are imperfection of technology that collected the data and the sources of the data itself [66]. Feature selection procedures select a subset of features from the original feature set without any transformation, maintaining the physical meanings of the original features and selecting those features that are capable of discriminating between the samples that belong to different classes.

Three main approaches are used for feature selection: filter, wrapper, and embedded. Filter methods use statistical feature properties to filter out irrelevant attributes. Wrapper methods explore the entire attribute space to score subsets of attributes based on their predictive power. Embedded methods attempt to find an optimal subset of features while constructing the predictive model at the same time [67].

Dimensionality reduction is one of the most popular techniques. It is used to select the features with less dimensionality, thus to improve the machine learning classifier generalization ability and accuracy while lowering the computational complexity. Principal Component Analysis (PCA) is a popular feature selection method in terms of dimensionality reduction. PCA is a linear combination of all the original variables; thus it is often difficult to interpret the results [68]. Alternatively, Lasso is a promising variable selection technique. It minimizes the residual sum of squares subject to the sum of the absolute value of the coefficients being less than a constant. Because of its nature, this constraint tends to produce some coefficients that are exactly 0 and hence gives interpretable sparse models which make it favorable as a variable selection method [69]. Another feature selection method is the Kruskal–Wallis test. It is a non-parametric one-way analysis of variance (ANOVA) test that is simple to implement and widely used in clinical data sets [70]. Another feature selection method is the linear mixed effect model (LME), which is a powerful and flexible tool used to reduce the feature set when we need to differentiate patients on a clinical scale. The LME models are based on a restricted maximum likelihood estimation method and have been widely used in medical diagnostics studies [71]. Other feature selection methods are Pearson and Spearman correlations, which are often used to assess the correlation between two variables. Pearson's correlation assesses the linear relationship, whereas Spearman's correlation assesses the monotonic relationship between variables. Chi-square also is one of the most effective methods for feature selection; it measures the degree of independence between the feature and the categories. It is also quite effective when the number of features is very small [72].

4.5.3 Classification algorithms

The main objective of the machine learning algorithms or classifications is to create patterns to describe, analyze, and predict data. These patterns are created from a set of examples, instances, composed of the extracted features [25]. Generally, there are three different kinds of machine learning algorithms: supervised, unsupervised, and reinforcement learning.

In supervised machine learning algorithms, the training of the pattern recognition systems is made by a set of labeled data; in unsupervised machine learning, the system is trained with unlabeled data. In reinforcement learning, the machine is trained to make a specific decision. The machine learns from past decisions and tries to determine the best possible solution according to the available and past knowledge [73]. Different machine learning algorithms are used in the area of AAL applications. Some commonly used algorithms are thresholding-based classifiers, neural networks, support vector machine (SVM), hidden Markov model, instance-based (K-nearest-neighbors), and probabilistic (Naïve Bayes (NB)).

Thresholding-based classifiers are often used in assisted living applications for the binary classification problem. They classify one of the two states based on the threshold. When the value of features is above the threshold, it will consider one state, and for feature value below the threshold, it is for the other state. Among these classifiers are decision trees (DT) and random forest (RF). Decision trees are widely used in recognition problems and are based on test questions and conditions. Each node represents a test; the branches represent outcomes, while the leaves are the final labels [25]. A random forest is made of a certain number of decision trees. Each tree gives a classification output, and the final output will be the maximum voting among the trees. Each tree is built on a vector of features built randomly from the starting ones [74].

Instance-based classifiers such as K-nearest neighbors make decisions based on the instance under test. These classifiers do not need training data, but they are computationally intensive.

Neural networks are basically human brain inspired classifiers generally used in deep learning for complex daily activities and also for clinical decision-making such as healthy or unhealthy. It consists of a large set of nodes with weighted connections. It can provide high classification accuracy with a large set of training data. However, typically in assisted living applications, a large set of training data often is not available, which make it less favorable in the assisted living applications [61].

SVM is a very popular classification algorithm often used in assisted living applications. SVM is unique among the other machine learning techniques because of its ability to distribute population in high-dimensional feature space. This algorithm was initially applied only to binary classification, finding the optimal separating hyperplane between two datasets. In a multiclass problem, a one-versus-one strategy is used to adopt SVM in multiclass problems [75]. SVM categorized the data based on the trained model by using a unique technique known as kernel. Different kinds of kernels can be found in advanced systems, including linear, polynomial, and radial basis function [76]. SVM does not need a large set for the training model, which is an advantage compared to neural networks [61].

HMM is the statistical Markov model, in which the system assumes the Markov process with unobserved hidden states. HMM can be presented as the simplest dynamic Bayesian network. HMM is often used in speech recognition and gesture recognition. It is commonly used in inertial measurement unit-based sensor data to recognize the daily activities and sequence of movements [61].

To compare the performances of the different classification algorithms and have a quantitative analysis of the results, different parameters can be evaluated beginning with the confusion matrix (i.e. accuracy, F-measure, precision, recall, and specificity, as described in [25]).

4.6 SensHand for recognizing daily gesture

This section presents a concrete application of gesture recognition based on wearable IMUs.

In this application, the SensHand was used to recognize nine different gestures typically performed in activities of daily living (eat some crackers with the hand (HA); drink from a glass (GL); eat some fruit with the fork (FK); eat some yogurt with a spoon (SP); drink from a cup (CP); answer the phone (PH); brush the teeth with a tooth brush (TB); brush the hair with a hair brush (HB); dry the hair with the hair dryer (HD)). The study consisted of different phases: in the first step, the attention was focused on finding the best combination of sensors that could recognize the gestures [77]. Then, the optimal solution was analyzed in greater depth to reduce the number of features to be used and use the new dataset as input for the machine learning algorithms.

Experimental setting

The SensHand was used for the acquisition, but the finger sensors were placed on the intermediate phalange of the index and middle finger instead of on the distal one. Data from accelerometers and gyroscopes were collected at 50 Hz, already filtered with a fourth-order low-pass digital filter with a cutoff frequency of 5 Hz. A more detailed description of the acquisition protocol can be found in [77].

Data Processing and Analysis

After the acquisition, the signals coming from the sensors were segmented according to the label to separate each gesture in the sequences. The complete dataset consisted of 7,200 gestures. Mean, standard deviation, root mean square, and MAD were extracted from each axis of the accelerometer.

As described in Moschetti *et al.* [77], two different machine learning algorithms, i.e., DT and SVM, were applied to find the best combination of sensors able to recognize the gestures. Two kinds of analysis were carried out, a personal analysis, where the same user was used as training and testing, and a leave-one-subject-out analysis (LOSO), where one participant was used as a test set on a model trained on the 19 participants. Results showed that the combination of sensors that use the index finger and the wrist sensors gave good results compared to other configurations. Using these two sensors provided excellent results in terms of accuracy and F-measure (0.89 and 0.884, respectively) while maintaining a low obtrusiveness for the users.

Starting from this configuration, further analyses were conducted. In particular, the data set was reduced. Considering the sensor on the wrist and the one on the index finger, our dataset was made of 7,200 gestures and 24 features. To remove the features that were too correlated, the Pearson correlation coefficient between each feature was computed, and the features with a coefficient greater than ± 0.85 were removed [78].

The new dataset is composed of 15 uncorrelated features. The matrix of the features was then normalized according to a Z-norm, to have zero mean and a unit standard deviation, to avoid distortion due to data heterogeneity.

To find similarity between gestures, for each gesture the mean values and the standard deviation were computed beginning with the reduced dataset. Then, PCA was applied to improve the visualization of the features in the principal component space. The standard deviation quantifies the variation in performing a specific gesture.

An SVM with a third-order polynomial kernel was applied to the features dataset to recognize the gestures and provide a quantitative analysis of the performances. A LOSO analysis was carried out to evaluate whether the system trained on 19 users was able to recognize the gestures performed by an unknown user. The system was trained leaving one user out, in turn, and then tested on the left-out subject. Then, a mean of the results was evaluated. This analysis was performed in Weka—Data Mining Suite [79].

Results

Results from previous work showed that using two sensors placed on the intermediate phalange of the finger and on the wrist allow recognition among nine gestures of daily living [77]. In this further analysis, a reduction of the features was computed, and a third-order polynomial kernel SVM was applied in a LOSO analysis to evaluate the performances of the system. Precision, recall, specificity, accuracy, and F-measure were computed to have a quantitative analysis of the performance.

The analysis showed good results in terms of accuracy and F-measure (0.9232 ± 0.05 and 0.9288 ± 0.05, respectively).

In Figure 4.4, the values for the precision, recall, and F-measure are reported for each gesture.

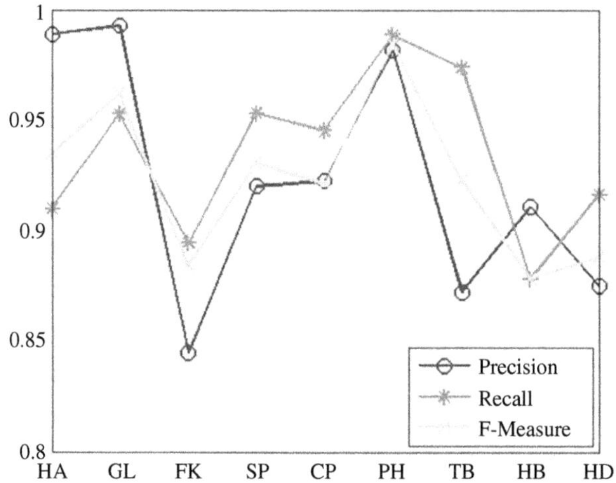

Figure 4.4 Values of precision, recall, and F-measure for each gesture

	HA	GL	FK	SP	CP	PH	TB	HB	HD
HA	791.0				9.0				
GL	3.0	794.0			3.0				
FK	30.0	6.0	676.0	46.0	41.0	1.0			
SP	1.0		52.0	737.0	10.0				
CP	9.0	50.0	1.0	1.0	738.0		1.0		
PH	13.0	1.0				785.0			1.0
TB	35.0					7.0	698.0	36.0	24.0
HB	10.0				1.0		10.0	728.0	51.0
HD						2.0	4.0	94.0	700.0

Figure 4.5 Confusion matrix for SVM model in the LOSO analysis for the entire dataset

Considering the F-measure of each gesture, FK and HB are the worst recognized gestures. Looking at the confusion matrix (Figure 4.5), it can be seen that the FK gesture is often confused with the SP one. The two gestures are often confused between each other due to the similarity of the movements. Other two gestures with a low F-measure with respect to the others are HB and HD. Even in this case, the confusion matrix shows how the two gestures are often mutually confused. In addition, the CP

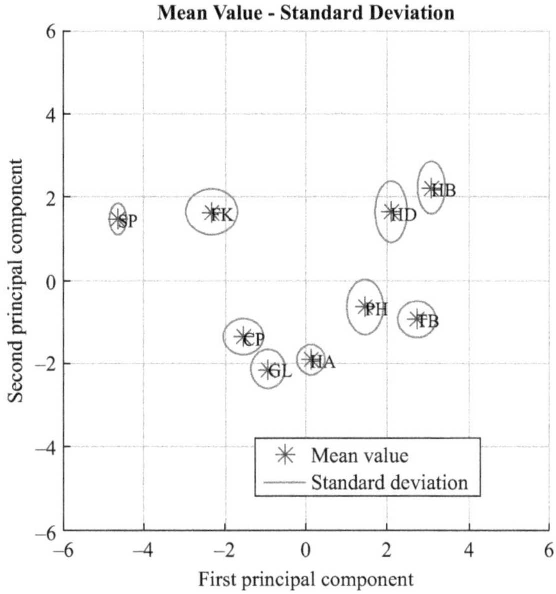

Figure 4.6 Mean gestures in the PCA-space

gesture does not reach a high value of F-measure, as it is often confused with GL. The highest values of F-measure are reached for HA, GL, and PH (all >0.94).

The same can be observed from the representation of the mean gestures in the PCA-space (Figure 4.6). In accordance with the variance, the first two principal components explain the 78.25% of the variance of the original dataset. HD and HB; PH and TB; and CP,GL and HA are very similar gestures, and sometimes they could be mutually confused, as shown in the confusion matrix. In Figure 4.6, it is also possible to observe how similarly the users performed the gestures. As a matter of fact, the circle around the star represents the standard deviation from the mean value representing the gestures. It can be seen that the SP gesture is the most precise gesture performed by the 20 users; the standard deviation has the lower values. On the contrary, FK and PH are the gestures which have greater variability, meaning that the users had performed the gestures in different ways.

These results showed that using a sensor on the index finger and a sensor on the wrist allows to recognize nine different gestures generally performed in activities of daily living. Recognizing these gestures could be useful to monitor persons during daily life, without being too obtrusive. As a matter of fact, at the moment, the SensHand was used to acquire the data, but further improvement could bring the development of a smart ring and smart bracelets, therefore decreasing the intrusiveness. The use of the same sensors could be further investigated to increase the number of gestures and thus activities to be recognized, and it could also be used to control robots and smart appliances.

4.7 Conclusion

According to the demographic projection, the number of elderly people will increase in the coming years, raising challenges to find new solutions to help them stay healthy and independent. AAL technologies can provide solutions to help older individuals stay longer in their own homes, monitored and supported, and to make them and their caregivers feel safe. As described in Section 4.3, gesture recognition can play an important role in the use of this technological solution.

In recent years, various technologies have been developed to recognize gestures, spanning from wearable sensors to video-based sensors. The choice of the device strongly depends on the application.

Considering the presented application, a few steps remain to bring these technologies into real life. In particular, regarding use of the SensHand for recognition of daily gestures, the next step will be to implement an online algorithm that will allow the sensor to be used in daily living, and be able to discriminate among different gestures. Moreover, other applications could be implemented so it can be used for training purposes as well. In addition, people can indeed perform exercises with this sensor while being at home, which will create a "*continuum of care*" and increase the rehabilitation hours, making it more efficient. However, further investigations should be performed to determine the most comfortable way to use the different technologies for all the patients, with low to advanced stages of disease.

Future developments will look toward the implementation of different applications using the same sensors. The use of a set of sensors at home for monitoring, training, and controlling smart appliances and devices would allow individuals to have a set of tools to be used in daily life. In a house with many AAL technologies, for instance, robots could be controlled and teleoperated to make them perform dangerous activities such as preventing people from falling and becoming injured. The same sensors could be used by the robot to perceive what the user is doing and the understand the non-verbal cues that people use to communicate, allowing a more natural interaction. At the same time, sensors can be used as monitoring tools both for clinicians in case of already existing diseases and also for checking daily habits and preventing degeneration of cognitive and physical abilities. Therefore, gesture recognition represents an important tool for several AAL applications.

References

[1] "Demography – trends and projections 2015, European Commission," http://ec.europa.eu/economy_finance/structural_reforms/ageing/demography/index_en.htm, accessed: 2016-11-21.

[2] D. I. Auerbach, "Will the np workforce grow in the future?: New forecasts and implications for healthcare delivery," *Medical Care*, vol. 50, no. 7, pp. 606–610, 2012.

[3] R. S. Hooker, J. F. Cawley, and C. M. Everett, "Predictive modeling the physician assistant supply: 2010–2025," *Public Health Reports*, vol. 126, no. 5, pp. 708–716, 2011.

[4] "Why Robots Are the Future of Elder Care, The Daily Good," https://www.good.is/articles/robots-elder-care-pepper-exoskeletons-japan, accessed: 2016-11-21.

[5] "Ambient Assisted Living Roadmap," http://www.aaliance2.eu/sites/default/files/AA2_WP2_D2%207_RM2_rev5.0.pdf, accessed: 2016-11-21.

[6] "Ambient Assisted Living Strategic Research Agenda," http://www.aaliance2.eu/sites/default/files/AA2_D2.7b_SRA2014_v4.0.pdf, accessed: 2016-11-21.

[7] D. J. Cook and N. C. Krishnan, *Activity Learning: Discovering, Recognizing, and Predicting Human Behavior from Sensor Data*. Hobokeb, NJ, John Wiley & Sons, 2015.

[8] R. Tarricone and A. D. Tsouros, *Home Care in Europe: The Solid Facts*. Milan, Italy: WHO Regional Office Europe, 2008.

[9] A. Moschetti, L. Fiorini, M. Aquilano, F. Cavallo, and P. Dario, "Preliminary findings of the aaliance2 ambient assisted living roadmap," in *Ambient Assisted Living*. Cham (ZG), Switzerland, Springer, 2014, pp. 335–342.

[10] G. van den Broek, F. Cavallo, and C. Wehrmann, *AALIANCE Ambient Assisted Living Roadmap*. Netherlands, Amsterdam, IOS Press, 2010, vol. 6.

[11] H. Yan, M. H. Ang Jr, and A. N. Poo, "A survey on perception methods for human–robot interaction in social robots," *International Journal of Social Robotics*, vol. 6, no. 1, pp. 85–119, 2014.

[12] S. L. Gorst, C. J. Armitage, S. Brownsell, and M. S. Hawley, "Home telehealth uptake and continued use among heart failure and chronic obstructive pulmonary disease patients: A systematic review," *Annals of Behavioral Medicine*, vol. 48, no. 3, pp. 323–336, 2014.

[13] "Medical Electronics Market – Global Forecast to 2022," http://www.marketsandmarkets.com/PressReleases/medical-electronics.asp, accessed: 2016-11-21.

[14] "Smart Home Market – Global Forecast to 2022," http://www.marketsandmarkets.com/Market-Reports/smart-homes-and-assisted-living-advanced-technologie-and-global-market-121.html, accessed: 2016-11-21.

[15] "Telehealth Market – Global Forecast to 2022," http://www.marketsandmarkets.com/PressReleases/telehealth.asp, accessed: 2016-11-21.

[16] "The advent of digital health," http://www.strategy-business.com/blog/The-Advent-of-Digital-Health?gko=f2f63, accessed: 2016-11-21.

[17] "Ericsson Mobility Report 2016," https://www.ericsson.com/res/docs/2016/ericsson-mobility-report-2016.pdf, accessed: 2016-11-24.

[18] "CSS Insight – Wearable Tech Market To Be Worth $34 Billion By 2019," http://www.ccsinsight.com/press/company-news/2332-wearables-market-to-be-worth-25-billion-by-2019-reveals-ccs-insight, accessed: 2016-11-24.

[19] N. K. Suryadevara, S. C. Mukhopadhyay, R. Wang, and R. Rayudu, "Forecasting the behavior of an elderly using wireless sensors data in a smart

home," *Engineering Applications of Artificial Intelligence*, vol. 26, no. 10, pp. 2641–2652, 2013.

[20] J. R. Napier, "The prehensile movements of the human hand," *Bone & Joint Journal*, vol. 38, no. 4, pp. 902–913, 1956.

[21] M. Gowing, A. Ahmadi, F. Destelle, D. S. Monaghan, N. E. O'Connor, and K. Moran, "Kinect vs. low-cost inertial sensing for gesture recognition," *International Conference on Multimedia Modeling*, Springer International Publishing, pp. 484–495, 2014.

[22] A. Ferrone, F. Maita, L. Maiolo, *et al.*, "Wearable band for hand gesture recognition based on strain sensors," in *2016 Sixth IEEE International Conference on Biomedical Robotics and Biomechatronics (BioRob)*. Singapore, IEEE, 2016, pp. 1319–1322.

[23] W. Lu, Z. Tong, and J. Chu, "Dynamic hand gesture recognition with leap motion controller," *IEEE Signal Processing Letters*, vol. 23, no. 9, pp. 1188–1192, 2016.

[24] S. Mitra and T. Acharya, "Gesture recognition: A survey," *IEEE Transactions on Systems, Man, and Cybernetics, Part C (Applications and Reviews)*, vol. 37, no. 3, pp. 311–324, 2007.

[25] O. D. Lara and M. A. Labrador, "A survey on human activity recognition using wearable sensors," *IEEE Communications Surveys & Tutorials*, vol. 15, no. 3, pp. 1192–1209, 2013.

[26] A. Moncada-Torres, K. Leuenberger, R. Gonzenbach, A. Luft, and R. Gassert, "Activity classification based on inertial and barometric pressure sensors at different anatomical locations," *Physiological Measurement*, vol. 35, no. 7, p. 1245, 2014.

[27] F. Cavallo, D. Esposito, E. Rovini, *et al.*, "Preliminary evaluation of SensHand v1 in assessing motor skills performance in Parkinson disease," in *IEEE International Conference on Rehabilitation Robotics (ICORR)*. Seattle, WA, IEEE, 2013, pp. 1–6.

[28] D. Esposito and F. Cavallo, "Preliminary design issues for inertial rings in ambient assisted living applications," in *2015 IEEE International Instrumentation and Measurement Technology Conference (I2MTC) Proceedings*. Pisa, Italy, IEEE, 2015, pp. 250–255.

[29] E. Rovini, D. Esposito, C. Maremmani, P. Bongioanni, and F. Cavallo, "Using wearable sensor systems for objective assessment of Parkinson's disease," in *20th IMEKO TC4 International Symposium and 18th International Workshop on ADC Modelling and Testing Research on Electric and Electronic Measurement for the Economic Upturn*, 2014, pp. 15–17.

[30] L. Dipietro, A. M. Sabatini, and P. Dario, "A survey of glove-based systems and their applications," *IEEE Transactions on Systems, Man, and Cybernetics, Part C (Applications and Reviews)*, vol. 38, no. 4, pp. 461–482, 2008.

[31] F. Parvini and C. Shahabi, "Utilizing bio-mechanical characteristics for user-independent gesture recognition," in *21st International Conference on Data Engineering Workshops (ICDEW'05)*. Washington DC, IEEE, 2005, pp. 1170–1170.

[32] M. A. Mohandes, "Recognition of two-handed Arabic signs using the cyberglove," *Arabian Journal for Science and Engineering*, vol. 38, no. 3, pp. 669–677, 2013.
[33] J.-W. Lin, C. Wang, Y. Y. Huang, *et al.*, "Backhand: Sensing hand gestures via back of the hand," in *Proceedings of the 28th Annual ACM Symposium on User Interface Software & Technology*. Charlotte, NC, ACM, 2015, pp. 557–564.
[34] S. Jin, Y. Li, G.-m. Lu, J.-x. Luo, W.-d. Chen, and X.-x. Zheng, "Som-based hand gesture recognition for virtual interactions," in *IEEE International Symposium on VR Innovation (ISVRI)*. Singapore, IEEE, 2011, pp. 317–322.
[35] T. Chouhan, A. Panse, A. K. Voona, and S. Sameer, "Smart glove with gesture recognition ability for the hearing and speech impaired," in *IEEE Global Humanitarian Technology Conference-South Asia Satellite (GHTC-SAS)*, Trivandrum, India, 2014, pp. 105–110.
[36] C. Rishikanth, H. Sekar, G. Rajagopal, R. Rajesh, and V. Vijayaraghavan, "Low-cost intelligent gesture recognition engine for audio-vocally impaired individuals," in *Global Humanitarian Technology Conference (GHTC), 2014 IEEE*. San Jose, CA, IEEE, 2014, pp. 628–634.
[37] N. Carbonaro, A. Greco, G. Anania, *et al.*, "Unobtrusive physiological and gesture wearable acquisition system: A preliminary study on behavioral and emotional correlations," *The First International Conference on Global Health Challenges*, October 21–26, Venice, Italy, pp. 88–92, 2012.
[38] T. D. Bui and L. T. Nguyen, "Recognizing postures in Vietnamese sign language with MEMS accelerometers," *IEEE Sensors Journal*, vol. 7, no. 5, pp. 707–712, 2007.
[39] J.-H. Kim, N. D. Thang, and T.-S. Kim, "3-d hand motion tracking and gesture recognition using a data glove," in *2009 IEEE International Symposium on Industrial Electronics*. Lausanne, Switzerland, IEEE, 2009, pp. 1013–1018.
[40] C. Amma, M. Georgi, and T. Schultz, "Airwriting: Hands-free mobile text input by spotting and continuous recognition of 3D-space handwriting with inertial sensors," in *16th IEEE International Symposium on Wearable Computers*, Newcastle, UK, 2012, pp. 52–59.
[41] J. Lei, Z. Yinghui, Z. Cheng, and W. Junbo, "A recognition method for one-stroke finger gestures using a MEMS 3D accelerometer," *IEICE Transactions on Information and Systems*, vol. 94, no. 5, pp. 1062–1072, 2011.
[42] L. Jing, Y. Zhou, Z. Cheng, and T. Huang, "Magic ring: A finger-worn device for multiple appliances control using static finger gestures," *Sensors*, vol. 12, no. 5, pp. 5775–5790, 2012.
[43] M.-C. Hsieh, Y.-H. Yen, and T.-Y. Sun, "Gesture recognition with two 3-axis accelerometers," in *IEEE International Conference on Consumer Electronics-Taiwan (ICCE-TW)*. Taipei, Taiwan, IEEE, 2014, pp. 239–240.
[44] M. Roshandel, A. Munjal, P. Moghadam, S. Tajik, and H. Ketabdar, "Multi-sensor based gestures recognition with a smart finger ring," in *International Conference on Human-Computer Interaction*. Heraklion, Crete, Greece, Springer, 2014, pp. 316–324.

[45] G. R. Naik and H. T. Nguyen, "Nonnegative matrix factorization for the identification of EMG finger movements: Evaluation using matrix analysis," *IEEE Journal of Biomedical and Health Informatics*, vol. 19, no. 2, pp. 478–485, 2015.

[46] P.-G. Jung, G. Lim, S. Kim, and K. Kong, "A wearable gesture recognition device for detecting muscular activities based on air-pressure sensors," *IEEE Transactions on Industrial Informatics*, vol. 11, no. 2, pp. 485–494, 2015.

[47] M. T. Wolf, C. Assad, M. T. Vernacchia, J. Fromm, and H. L. Jethani, "Gesture-based robot control with variable autonomy from the JPL BioSleeve," in *IEEE International Conference on Robotics and Automation (ICRA)*. Karlsruhe, Germany, IEEE, 2013, pp. 1160–1165.

[48] Z. Lu, X. Chen, Q. Li, X. Zhang, and P. Zhou, "A hand gesture recognition framework and wearable gesture-based interaction prototype for mobile devices," *IEEE Transactions on Human-Machine Systems*, vol. 44, no. 2, pp. 293–299, 2014.

[49] M. Georgi, C. Amma, and T. Schultz, "Recognizing hand and finger gestures with IMU based motion and EMG based muscle activity sensing," in *Proceedings of the International Conference on Bio-inspired Systems and Signal Processing*, Lisbon, Portugal, 2015, pp. 99–108.

[50] I. Staretu and C. Moldovan, "Leap motion device used to control a real anthropomorphic gripper," *International Journal of Advanced Robotic Systems*, vol. 13, no. 3, p. 113, 2016.

[51] C. Alabart Gutiérrez del Olmo, "Study and analysis of the leap motion sensor and the software development kit (SDK) for the implementation of visual human computer interfaces," Degree Project 2015. Available at Archivo Digital UPM http://oa.upm.es/37299/

[52] G. Bieber, M. Haescher, and M. Vahl, "Sensor requirements for activity recognition on smart watches," in *Proceedings of the Sixth International Conference on PErvasive Technologies Related to Assistive Environments*. Island of Rhodes, Greece, ACM, 2013, p. 67.

[53] J. Rekimoto, "Gesturewrist and gesturepad: Unobtrusive wearable interaction devices," in *Proceedings of the Fifth IEEE International Symposium on Wearable Computers*, Zurich, Switzerland, 2001, pp. 21–27.

[54] D. J. Wile, R. Ranawaya, and Z. H. Kiss, "Smart watch accelerometry for analysis and diagnosis of tremor," *Journal of Neuroscience Methods*, vol. 230, pp. 1–4, 2014.

[55] K. Liu, C. Chen, R. Jafari, and N. Kehtarnavaz, "Multi-HMM classification for hand gesture recognition using two differing modality sensors," in *2014 IEEE Circuits and Systems Conference (DCAS)*, Dallas, IEEE, 2014, pp. 1–4.

[56] V. Ahanathapillai, J. D. Amor, Z. Goodwin, and C. J. James, "Preliminary study on activity monitoring using an android smart-watch," *Healthcare Technology Letters*, vol. 2, no. 1, pp. 34–39, 2015.

[57] H. Mousavi Hondori and M. Khademi, "A review on technical and clinical impact of Microsoft Kinect on physical therapy and rehabilitation," *Journal of Medical Engineering*, vol. 2014, pp. 16, 2014.

[58] S. Deterding, D. Dixon, R. Khaled, and L. Nacke, "From game design elements to gamefulness: Defining gamification," in *Proceedings of the 15th International Academic MindTrek Conference: Envisioning Future Media Environments*. Tampere, Finland, ACM, 2011, pp. 9–15.

[59] K.-H. Chen, P.-C. Lin, Y.-J. Chen, B.-S. Yang, and C.-H. Lin, "Development of method for quantifying essential tremor using a small optical device," *Journal of Neuroscience Methods*, vol. 266, pp. 78–83, 2016.

[60] N. Hosseinpour, "ICT in health-care," Master Thesis, Sweden, Gothenburg, Spring 2016. Available at http://publications.lib.chalmers.se/records/fulltext/241186/241186.pdf

[61] T. R. Bennett, J. Wu, N. Kehtarnavaz, and R. Jafari, "Inertial measurement unit-based wearable computers for assisted living applications: A signal processing perspective," *IEEE Signal Processing Magazine*, vol. 33, no. 2, pp. 28–35, 2016.

[62] M. Shoaib, S. Bosch, O. D. Incel, H. Scholten, and P. J. Havinga, "Fusion of smartphone motion sensors for physical activity recognition," *Sensors*, vol. 14, no. 6, pp. 10146–10176, 2014.

[63] Z. Zhang, Q. Fang, and X. Gu, "Objective assessment of upper-limb mobility for poststroke rehabilitation," *IEEE Transactions on Biomedical Engineering*, vol. 63, no. 4, pp. 859–868, 2016.

[64] E. Rovini, D. Esposito, C. Maremmani, P. Bongioanni, and F. Cavallo, "Empowering patients in self-management of Parkinson's disease through cooperative ICT systems," *Optimizing Assistive Technologies for Aging Populations*, p. 251, 2015.

[65] Y. S. Morsi, *Optimizing Assistive Technologies for Aging Populations*. IGI Global, 2015.

[66] J. Tang, S. Alelyani, and H. Liu, "Feature selection for classification: A review," *Data Classification: Algorithms and Applications*, p. 37, 2014. CRC Press, 2013, Available at https://pdfs.semanticscholar.org/310e/a531640728702fce6c743c1dd680a23d2ef4.pdf

[67] S. Maldonado, R. Montoya, and R. Weber, "Advanced conjoint analysis using feature selection via support vector machines," *European Journal of Operational Research*, vol. 241, no. 2, pp. 564–574, 2015.

[68] H. Zou, T. Hastie, and R. Tibshirani, "Sparse principal component analysis," *Journal of Computational and Graphical Statistics*, vol. 15, no. 2, pp. 265–286, 2006.

[69] R. Tibshirani, "Regression shrinkage and selection via the lasso," *Journal of the Royal Statistical Society. Series B (Methodological)*, pp. 267–288, 1996.

[70] S. Ali Khan, A. Hussain, A. Basit, and S. Akram, "Kruskal–Wallis-based computationally efficient feature selection for face recognition," *The Scientific World Journal*, vol. 2014, pp. 6, 2014.

[71] B. Winter, "Linear models and linear mixed effects models in R with linguistic applications," *arXiv preprint arXiv:1308.5499*, Aug. 2013. Available at https://arxiv.org/abs/1308.5499.

[72] X. Geng, T.-Y. Liu, T. Qin, and H. Li, "Feature selection for ranking," in *Proceedings of the 30th Annual International ACM SIGIR Conference on Research and Development in Information Retrieval*. Amsterdam, ACM, 2007, pp. 407–414.
[73] C. Elkan, "Evaluating classifiers," 2012. Available at http://cseweb.ucsd.edu/∼ elkan/250Bwinter 2012/classifiereval.pdf (Accessed on 10 March 2015).
[74] Z. Feng, L. Mo, and M. Li, "A random forest-based ensemble method for activity recognition," in *2015 37th Annual International Conference of the IEEE Engineering in Medicine and Biology Society (EMBC)*. Milan, Italy, IEEE, 2015, pp. 5074–5077.
[75] R. Begg and J. Kamruzzaman, "A machine learning approach for automated recognition of movement patterns using basic, kinetic and kinematic gait data," *Journal of Biomechanics*, vol. 38, no. 3, pp. 401–408, 2005.
[76] G. Rescio, A. Leone, and P. Siciliano, "Supervised expert system for wearable MEMS accelerometer-based fall detector," *Journal of Sensors*, vol. 2013, pp. 11, 2013.
[77] A. Moschetti, L. Fiorini, D. Esposito, P. Dario, and F. Cavallo, "Recognition of daily gestures with wearable inertial rings and bracelets," *Sensors*, vol. 16, no. 8, p. 1341, 2016.
[78] F. Attal, S. Mohammed, M. Dedabrishvili, F. Chamroukhi, L. Oukhellou, and Y. Amirat, "Physical human activity recognition using wearable sensors," *Sensors*, vol. 15, no. 12, pp. 31314–31338, 2015.
[79] M. Hall, E. Frank, G. Holmes, B. Pfahringer, P. Reutemann, and I. H. Witten, "The Weka data mining software: An update," *ACM SIGKDD explorations newsletter*, vol. 11, no. 1, pp. 10–18, 2009.

Chapter 5

Design and prototyping of an innovative home automation system for the monitoring of elderly people

Adriano Mancini, Emanuele Frontoni, Ilaria Ercoli, Rama Pollini, Primo Zingaretti, and Annalisa Cenci

Abstract

The population of elderly people keeps increasing rapidly. It is becoming a predominant aspect of our societies. It is therefore necessary to find ways to ensure the care of the needs of older people.

We propose the project AngelHome, an innovative home automation system for Ambient Assisted Living that aims to improve the lives of people in their homes. In this way they can live independently and safely within their home without changing their habits.

Angel Home offers an integrated and cooperative system with sensors and SOs to enhance the comfort inside the home. It also allows to ensure the safety people through the use of systems able to detect emergency situations.

Another objective of this project is the identification and classification of rare events, through machine learning approach, based on data coming from different embedded systems and from the information system. This amount of information (located in a cloud system) also enhances the intelligence of the house, which will learn from what happened in the past.

5.1 Introduction

Particularly in the last years, in the industrialized countries, the society is evolving toward an important demographic changing also known as the ageing society. This aspect is due to the increasing life expectancy, which causes the ageing of population. For this purpose, it is important to find innovative, productive and cheap solutions in order to maintain the expenses for the health care within the limits of economic possibility [1,2]. In this way, it is ensured a comfortable and dignified life for all older people who want to independently live in their home environment. Taking into account the studies of the World Health Organization [3], elderly people (people of

60 years of age and older) in the world are about 650 million and by 2050 will reach the 2 billion. This also happen for European population that will keep on growing older. In 2008 the population over the age of 65 was over 17 per cent, and in 2060 it will rise to 30 per cent, instead, the population over the age of 85 will go from 4 per cent to 12 per cent [4].

Considering this trend, it is important to implement smart solutions for elderly care since they should remain independent and able to work for a longer time. This can be achieved owing to the technology. In this context, Ambient Assisted Living (AAL) applications are placed that have attracted a growing attention in scientific community since they involve emerging and innovative technological solutions, providing embedded systems in the domestic environment. The principal aim of AAL is to increase the quality of life, reducing costs for independent living [5–8]. This, in order to enhance the self-confidence and autonomy of elderly or ill people and in the same time to increase security and avoid dangerous situations.

In this context, we propose the AngelHome project that aims to make better the life of older people and people with some disabilities ensuring their independence in their familiar and domestic environment.

In general, the home becomes smart, interacts with people and executes commands given but could also able to independently act, as in cases of emergency where for example a person falls on the floor [9–11] or when the presence of smoke is detected. Targeted actions are immediately triggered to ensure the safety of people and speed the arrival of relief supplies. In their home, older people better live, have more certainty, maintain contact with a known environment, keeping intact their world.

The aim of the project is to propose an innovative idea of an interoperable embedded intelligent system where different low cost smart sensors can analyze the human behaviors to obtain interactivity and statistical data, mainly oriented to Human Behavior Analysis (HBA) in intelligent AAL environments [7]. In literature are applied different technologies that use visual sensors (both RGB and RGBD) for people tracking and interaction analysis, where depth information has been used to evaluate users activity in different indoor environments [12–14]. An important part, preliminary to the development of the project, was the psycho cognitive analysis, where a sample of elderly people has been interviewed about their lifestyle and their knowledge and use of technology. So, in design phase, the Smart Objects have been designed and developed taking into account their answers in the given questionnaire.

The closely related concepts of Ambient Intelligence (AmI) [15–17] and AAL have provided a vision of the information society where the attention is directed toward the users, more efficient support services, enrichment opportunities for the user, and an optimized support for human interactions. Nowadays, people are surrounded by smart and intuitive interfaces, integrated in every kind of objects and environments [18]. The characteristics of an intelligent environment, in accordance with the users that use it, should be in general those listed below: not intrusive, personalized, adaptive and predictive. The introduction of smart environments offers new possibilities of integration but at the same time opens new challenges in terms of access to products and services by persons with disabilities [19–21]. The aspects related to accessibility are not yet well defined, since future guidelines for the development of the information society are still open, below different aspects: (1) type of technologies used to build new smart environments; (2) type and nature of new emergent applications and services; (3) different contexts of use which will extend the information society; and (4) strategies put in place to extend the use to all potential users. However, it seems increasingly clear that the accessibility and usability within smart environments by users with various features and requirements cannot be achieved with ad-hoc solutions.

The AngelHome project is linked to the Internet of Things (IoT) paradigm [22–24], where objects become smart, are localized, can acquire data, process and exchange them. Smart home and building applications [25,26] are particularly important for IoT scenario, as they represent the link between the individual (citizen, consumer) and the overlying layers of adoption of IoT paradigm (Smart City, Smart Grid). Actually, there is not a sufficiently evolved market of AAL for elderly and disabled users, as well as for AmI, with the consequent difficulty to forecast quantitative and qualitative aspects of request in these areas. The effectiveness in the use of living spaces and their technological systems is then assigned to the design capacity of integration between the physical characteristics and performance of the same spaces, supporting technologies that interact with them. This, in order to improve accessibility, safety, sustainable energy of the environments and their comfort, by treating and developing technologically advanced solutions in the following main areas of intervention and related development objectives: assistance, inclusion, security, well-being and comfort. Security is an important aspect, since a system has not only provide the traditional alarm system, but also has to control the activities of the users, as well as intrusion detection using the latest technologies (face recognition, presence of movement, sound identification). This security aspect is divided into instantaneous and adaptive.

The system for AAL applications has a high degree of integration with basic home automation functions and is interfaced with the most common home automation standards and their recent innovations.

5.2 General description of the Angel Home system

The objectives of the Angel Home project are to build a system that meets certain characteristics: monitoring of comfort and behavior of vulnerable persons/the elderly within the home, collection process and data processing, ability to interact with the outdoor and sending alarm management The system provides an inference engine (using deductive procedures) able to deduce conclusions based on the initial experience and knowledge gained during the execution (self-learning). In this context it is analyzed and studied a distributed monitoring system taking into account certain issues:

- Define who are the players in the system.
- Transpose data from the assisted housing: personal data, collected data from Smart Object (SO).

- Deal with the possible absence of connectivity between home and the Central System.
- Define of the alarms: severity/aging.
- Data presentation mode: Plans, Charts, Tables.
- Interdependencies between monitored objects.

It was defined an architecture that concentrates the data from the various houses in remote servers and capable of providing technology and interfaces for analysis and study of the data collected. Each house is equipped with numerous SmartObjects able to study the behavior and movements of the weak or elderly person (SmartTv and SmartCam) and be able to analyze and adjust the degree perceived comfort (environmental SmartSensors), in order to improve the way of life also in the presence of reduced mental capacity.

5.2.1 Architecture of the system

The architecture of Angel project can be divided into two main areas (Figure 5.1): The "Domotic House" characterized by SOs that collect data on patients and the "Data Center" that represents the heart of the system, consisting of many servers that

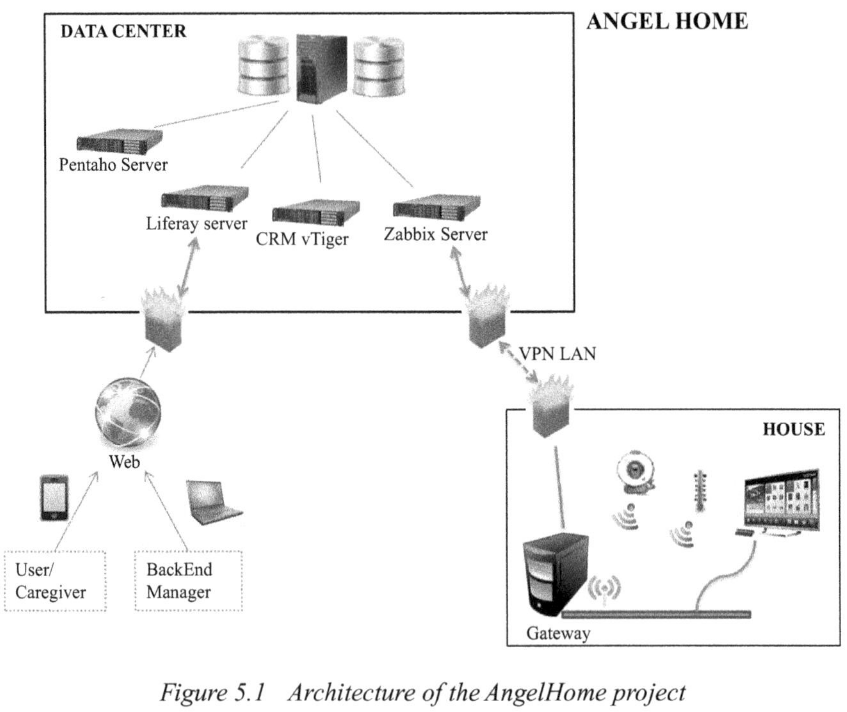

Figure 5.1 Architecture of the AngelHome project

perform activities management and data storage from housing and alert generation. The "Data Center" consists of:

- Vtiger CRM: has been customized to ensure effective management of the entities of an AAL project. For each home is managed the registry of the dwelling, tenant/assisted and SO installed. It was implemented a ticketing system for the processing of requests. A call or texting involves opening a ticket in which is associated with the reason for the request, the assisted contacts available and the priority of the request. The system is able to create tickets from sms/text messages automatically generated by alert internal to a dwelling.
- Zabbix: is based on a monitoring system that concentrates all the raw data from the SOs of different domestic environments.
- Pentaho: is a tool that enables the system to unify and manipulate data from different sources. It ensures the uniqueness and consistency of the data.
- Liferay portal: is a CMS platform that has the purpose of aggregating resources and provide services. It acts as a concentrator of data from the Vtiger CRM and the Zabbix server. It offers services for the creation of new house, allowing you to create objects "Dwelling", "Tenant/assisted", "Smart Objects", "Alarm", via a data entry coupled to an automatic data collection.

The entire architecture is integrated with a Single Sign ON-based system based on CAS (Central Authentication Server). The communication channel between the "Data Center" and the home automation housing is protected by VPN (Virtual Private Network) that guarantees security and robustness to data transmission.

The main stakeholders that interact with the system are:

- User/Caregiver: interacting with the MS using TV, smartphone and Web. Relatives of the elderly and caregivers receive alerts (by phone and SMS) when there is a problem with the patient.
- BackEnd Manager: Deals with monitoring the status of SO and network infrastructure. Implements the HBA using the data stored in the time.

5.2.2 Gateway description

The gateway provides the necessary services to the connection of SMs used within the Angel Home context, in order to ensure interoperability. The SMs operate with different communication protocols, either standard or proprietary, on wireless and wired channels, and even at the data-link layer. The gateway is able to manage the information coming from the various devices even in absence of a supervisor PC. It consists of two macro-blocks:

- Main Unit: constituted by a IMx-6 platform, used to manage and perform high-level and computationally onerous operations, since it has a high capacity of calculation. The main units offers several wired and wireless communication interfaces: 1 Gigabit Ethernet ports, two USB 2.0 ports, a Wi-Fi 802.11 and serial ports as RS232/RS422/RS485 interface. The main unit must reprocess data coming from the secondary drive.

- Secondary Unit: is realized as an active component and equipped with a low-performance microcontroller (k60 microcontroller). It is responsible for managing operations of the lowest level. Another task of secondary units is the interaction with the home SO. The communication of the secondary unit with combined primary and manufactured by one of the two RS232 ports. The unit constitutes an additional front of expandability in respect of the smart devices taken into account in the context of AngelHome.

5.2.3 Monitoring system: Zabbix

Zabbix is an open source monitoring software that allows to monitor the availability and performance of an IT infrastructure. The architecture is server-agent type, data can be collected through any type of device (server, network device, virtual machine) and can be defined rules that allows to generate alarms. Supports monitoring through data polling or by pushing/trapping can take advantage of the agent software available for all major operating systems or rely entirely on agent-less methods (SNMP, SSH, WMI, IPMI) to cover virtually any type of device. It allows to generate real-time graphics with instant alerts. The proposal in the new AngelHome project is to exploit Zabbix as the SO monitoring system inside the house. Figure 5.2 describes the exchange of data that occurs between the zabbix server (located in the data center) and the gateway within a dwelling. The main functions of the Zabbix server maintenance, delivery and management of alerts from gateway.

The SMs are connected (via different connection types) to the gateway which acts as a central home control. Then it is up to the gateway to communicate with

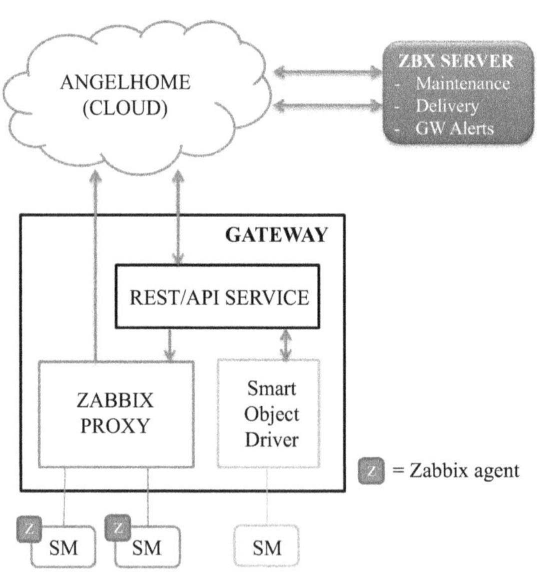

Figure 5.2 Communication system between Zabbix server and gateway

the outside of the house (the cloud). The gateway can be divided into three main parts:

- Zabbix Proxy: combines all monitoring data sent by the "Zabbix Agen". The Zabbix agent are demons that allow to communicate (actively or passively) with the Proxy by sending the information of changes in the state of SM monitored.
- SO Driver: Not all SOs are compatible to accommodate one "Zabbix agent" then the gateway provides the ability to install specific drivers so as to establish communication with the server.
- Rest/APi Service: is a module that provides rest/soap services to allow SMs to be able to communicate with Zabbix server without the help of Zabbix Proxy. This module increases the degree of AngelHome system interoperability.

5.3 Analysis and development of an automatic system for comfort control in the home

In domestic environments, the comfort control system is often entrusted to a central sensor that works on adjusting air temperature. This type of management leads to environments with a low level of comfort, which can lead to outbreaks of diseases in addition to an unpleasant perception of the environment. The state of modern interior air-conditioning systems allows to achieve excellent levels of indoor climate control, operating a simultaneous control over several parameters simultaneously. To the value of the ambient temperature, other parameters are associated, such as the mean radiant temperature, air velocity and relative humidity. These parameters are then mixed in order to arrive at the calculation of the PMV (Predicted Mean Vote) as a synthetic indicator of environmental quality. In addition to these parameters we added the Indoor Air Quality parameters: at first sight it comes to CO_2 content (related to air quality) and detection of CO (tied to the user's safety in the home). The CO_2 and CO parameters trigger alarms of varying severity that allow the user to operate an immediate fix. It has also been considered an environmental noise parameter linked to the passive acoustic requirements that a domestic environment must be able to give. The data have to be interpreted to express an opinion on the domestic environment to define its suitability for weaker user presence, to his health and even his ability to interact with the corrective indications that the system provides.

5.3.1 SmartSensor List

The list of sensors are: the ambient temperature, mean radiant temperature, the moisture content, radiant asymmetry, vertical temperature gradient, floor temperature, air speed. We added also parameters related to indoor air quality: the presence of harmful substances (VOC), CO_2 level, CO level.

A corollary of all this introduces an acoustic nature disorder linked to the noise of the environment and the internal environment noise (related to the respect of passive acoustic requirements of building and then sanitary requirement). The aim of the work is to store enough data to reach the global parameter of comfort required by UNI 7730.

Table 5.1 Environmental parameters given in Regulation 7730

Category	Thermal state of the body as a whole		Local discomfort			
	PPD %	PMV	DR %	PD % caused by		
				Vertical difference of air temperature	Hot or cold floor	Radiant asymmetry
A	<6	$-0.2 < PMV < +0.2$	<10	<3	<10	<5
B	<10	$-0.5 < PMV < +0.5$	<20	<5	<10	<5
C	<15	$-0.7 < PMV < +0.7$	<30	<10	<15	<10

These values will be saved in historical series and will compete to the calculation of the PMV as a synthetic indicator of environmental quality. The value of the PMV, the dimensionless value, should be kept within a very narrow range: $-0.5 < PMV < 0.5$. The permanence outside of this range will be signaled standardized and must be implemented an appropriate correction. Such a situation would indicate a situation of progressive distancing from such dangerous health conditions for health as more distant than the reference (0 value of PMV). Table 5.1 shows the comfort category with which the living environment is classified. The study of the performance of the reference class is an indicator on imported housing unit run.

The PPD (Percentage of Persons Dissatisfied) is another index defined in the ISO 7730 standard which allows to describe the percentage of dissatisfied people in a given environment. The PMV and PPD indices give an indication of comfort based on average values of environmental variables that define the "global comfort". It is also necessary to be aware of possible non-uniformity of the environmental variables caused by unwanted localized heating or cooling in the body. Two variables can be distinguished:

- DR (Risk Draft): is the percentage of people who perceive discomfort due to drafts localized (turbulence)
- PD (People Dissatisfied): is the percentage of people dissatisfied due to the vertical difference of air temperature, hot or cold floor or due to the asymmetry in the thermal exchanges by radiation (radiant asymmetry).

Concerning the air quality must keep in mind that the inspired air contains 21 per cent oxygen and 0.035 per cent of carbon dioxide. The expired air, however, contains only 16 per cent oxygen, but already the 4 per cent of carbon dioxide. The carbon dioxide is toxic to humans at a concentration of 2.5 per cent, but already starting from a concentration of 0.08 per cent (800 ppm) of carbon dioxide performance, concentration and well-being are compromised. To get an air quality will be verified compliance with the 1,000 ppm CO_2 limit.

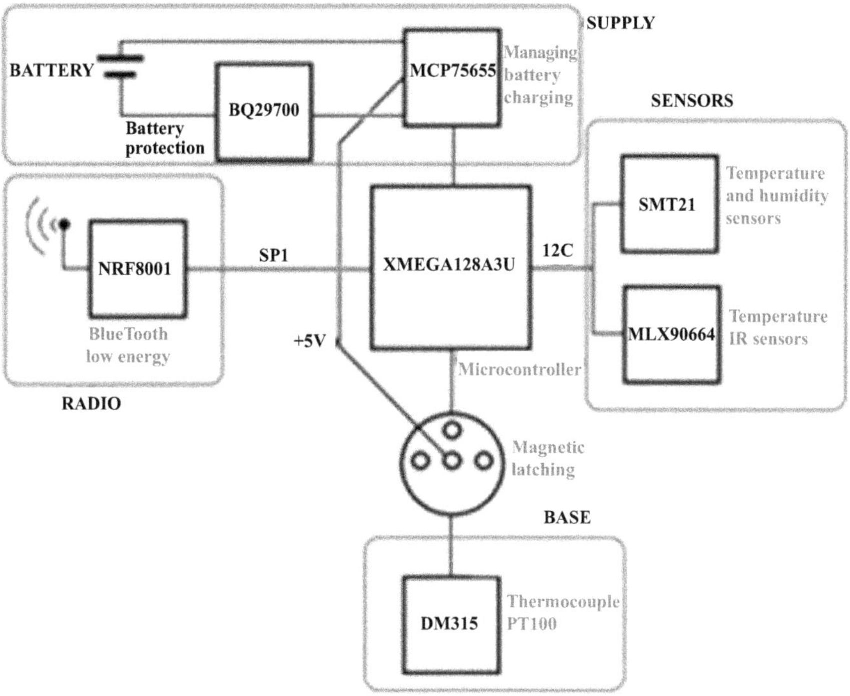

Figure 5.3 BTLEsensor

5.3.2 Smart Sensors: prototyping

For reasons relating to energy saving, the sensor has been divided into two parts, one part remains mobile and wireless as the original design (BTLEsensor). The other becomes a fixed base (USBsensor) that also serves as a gate for the collection of data BTLEsensor. Figure 5.3 describes the BTLEsensor while Figure 5.4 describes the USBsensor.

During the implementation of BTLEsensor, one of the aspects that have been most thorough was the energy savings. Appropriate changes to the card in order to lengthen the battery life were made, one of the main measures was to use the crystal oscillator as a reference for putting on standby the whole board and then turn it back on at regular intervals to take measurements and send them via bluetooth to USBsensor.

5.3.3 Testing in a controlled environment

It was experienced the subsystem for the analysis of the thermo hygrometric comfort and the healthiness of the air in real indoor environment. For the testing phase a domestic environment has been chosen. The main rooms where the unit and the respective sensors satellites positioned are the bedroom, the kitchen-dining area and

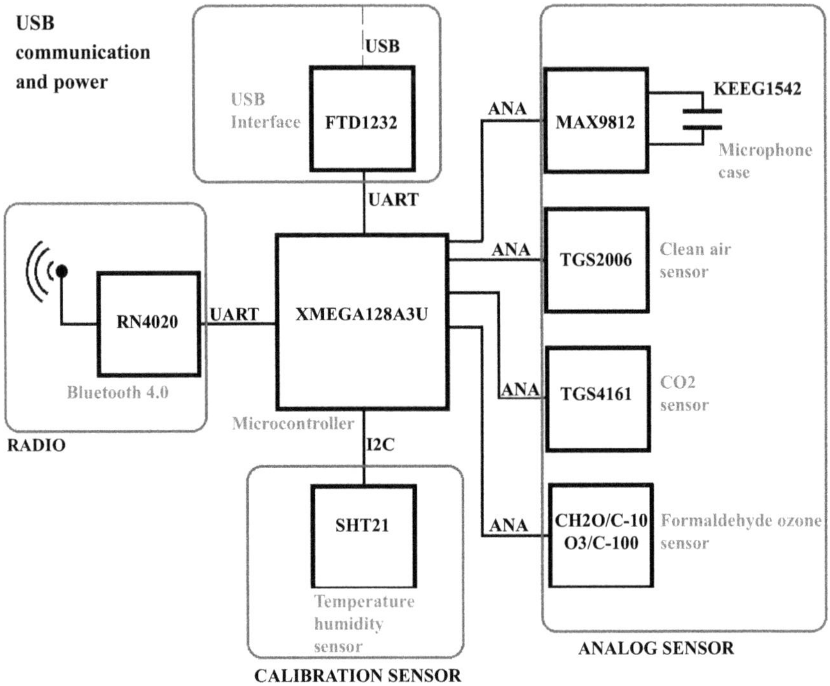

Figure 5.4 USBsensor

bathroom. For the selection of data acquisition neighboring points with the external walls of the dwelling and in particular those points most at risk of mold and condensation phenomena (form thermal bridges, walls weakly irradiated) have been privileged. The place was known the conditions of use of the occupants based on a repetition in the time scale of a single day in that week. This was necessary to allow the interpretation of data collected as much as possible consistent with the actual environmental situations, which have produced them. In this work, has been very helpful support provided by the occupants of the spaces in question have noted through various information questionnaire: use-programming of the heating or cooling; on–off, prolonged use of hot water in the bathroom and signaling of situations of discomfort at the time when these were perceived. The test phase lasts for about a month. The historical data were collected and analyzed on a weekly basis. In a real considered environment, it has been verified as the subsystem is able to 'tell' what is happening in the environment in terms of use and therefore the variations of the environmental parameters as a result of these. The recorded data historians have shown a congruence between the exceeding of the limit parameters set by ISO 7730 and the known behavior of the occupants or the use and programming of the air conditioning system. The major limitation found in this phase is given by the arc time used for the analysis of the behavior of the subsystem, circumscribed to a few weeks, limited to the winter season and then that was able to provide only a partial verification of the subsystem for the foreseeable internal situations and analyzable.

5.4 Psycho cognitive analysis

A technological system for the elderly must include the study and development of interfaces that allow to optimize the communication among these users. The research was necessary because there is currently no systematic report and it is clear that the interface should also take into account the complexity due to the context in which older people live. This research is fundamental because this is, for the older people, a completely new experience of communication that needs to be nearly their inclination. We are convinced that only in this way the AAL technologies could be accepted. The interview has been drafted in stages until reaching a model that would allow to researchers to acquire as much data and information as possible on the health report for those in primary beneficiaries of assistance, of their relationship with technology, some references to the dynamics cognitive, useful for computer graphics interface design of AAL and finally the perception that caregivers of their clients and the possible relationship of these with technology, and the way in which technological devices can be useful in everyday life. With data collection (all the results with the research methodology are available), the researchers went on to identify the lifestyles of the male respondents and female residents in the country and between the ages of 75 and 89 years. From these interviews it is emerged that the lifestyles of the people of this age group are mainly of two types: (a) sedentary for those who live in large cities, medium-large and (b) people who live in small towns, urban neighborhoods – due to the need to find primary and secondary livelihoods – alternate pet stay with acquaintances in the environment of urban places (supermarkets, parks, gardens, markets, small shops and social clubs). In both cases (a) and (b) the domestic environment in which the person resides and carries out most of the household activities coincides with the room where there is the television that is the kitchen, the living room. The analysis of the interviewee's answer shows like today the knowledge of technology, for the 40 per cent of older people, is declined with the use of TV, telephone/cell phone. Only the 30 per cent of them also speaks of pocket video games used by grandchildren. In addition, although many have undergone surgical operations, almost all of the subjects tend not to mention technological instruments used for medical use, this aspect of a certain importance. Few cases where it is reported the use of technologies for medical purposes in a domestic environment (30 per cent). The senior from an AAL device would on the one hand an aid for its domestic and relational activities (birthdays, bill payments, medical appointments, meetings, special holidays), and other support to the physiological critical without invading too some aspects of the subject of intimacy ensuring this certain degree of autonomy in their home environment. In the case in which a device requires a strong interaction with the end user – as for this AAL – the relationship between graphics and cognitive response is very narrow. The family uses some gesture that can be implemented to communicate with the device helps the user himself in understanding the cognitive effort that is required by the device based on the achievement of a task. Fundamental, in this research, in addition to the differentiation of linguistic repertoires of verbal and non, attitudes, thinking patterns, the influence exerted by changes of communication tools occurred in the course of time. This study is very important because the elderly – who has met the digital communication system in adulthood, after using for a long time traditional systems – interacts, within the project, with technological devices and being a great service user, he lives various experiences of communicative relations. Today the word "new technology" alarms the old person, and this made their experienced difficulties. So the first step is not to depart from the existent since there are people who cannot get used to the new, or who simply have no interest in the various functions of the devices. We need to develop a feeling of trust in the device so as to decrease anxiety and increase self-esteem of the person. At the same time, it should be avoided denial of verbalization of needs that aggravate the psychic fragmentation. Going specifically, device may refer to a technological support that, by using a screen to communicate with the client (such as that of a tablet or of a television), is able to activate an elderly alert through the issuance of well audible sounds irrespective of the volume used and repeated at least a couple of times. The sound should be able to be accompanied by a short text that indicates why the view and which can conduct the subject should be adopted. The message text must be written with a medium to large character, with a kerning (distance between one point and another) greater than that suggested by default by the program you are using to build the interface. Always on the part linked to cognitive processes, according to respondents, and the red caregiver appears to be one that attracts attention. Identified the daily activities of the subjects, their predisposition toward new technologies and how these can be used in everyday life we proceeded with the identification of the behaviors that the devices may have to communicate with beneficiaries of assistance and its interaction with the support. Asked how are technological devices should report to people the things to do? In most cases, individuals respond with a sound while someone responds "I do not know". While wondering about the usefulness of having a single device with more features or more devices with a single function, almost all respondents (95 per cent) answered "a single device with multiple functions". Going to stimulus that the device could produce, respondents suggest sounds, colourful signs, written associated with sound. The text is important because, according to the subjects, it helps to understand what the sound relates. It is preferable that the signal is repeated several times.

5.5 Analysis and implementation of a monitoring system of the user's physical and psychological behaviors weak (SmartCam and SmartTv)

At this stage of the AngelHome project was implemented a system to evaluate the evolution of mental decline, even with the prospect of being able to diagnose, in advance, any diseases that fall outside the natural process of dementia. It therefore considers it essential to rethink a new housing solution for the elderly, appropriately organized and as to provide all the information suited, to take the appropriate decisions to evaluate when a person is no longer able to live alone. The dementia syndrome occurs gradually from a mild cognitive impairment and can develop with slow deterioration, such as to involve a period of several years, or in a manner progressive, in the short term. Identify dementia at an early stage can be crucial to start the search for a cause possibly treatable or, at least, able to delay the hospitalization of the subject in a specialized structure. In order to achieve the purpose described above two SOs have been implemented: (1) SmartTv and (2) SmartCam (smart camera). Both tools allow to monitor, in a different way, users behavior weakness in their home. By crossing the information from the two SOs it can get an overview of the possible user's mental decay monitored. Another in-depth look in this project was to leverage machine learning approach [27] to automate the process of detection of behaviors that can be traced to a deterioration of the patient's mental processes.

5.5.1 SmartCam

The purpose of the project is achieved through the implementation of a system able to acquire and process at all times images of the individual concerned and the environment in which it operates. This means putting in place a constant diagnosis system and invisible from the monitored subject, extremely more effective than human control that, as accurate, may not be able to judge the small behavioral changes of the subject, with the risk to intervene when the disease has now reached an advanced stage and therefore no longer curable. The SmartCam placed in the rooms of the system allow to analyze the habits regarding the places where the monitored subject spends more time and is capable of general alerts when changes arise. The SmartCam captures images at predefined intervals [28].

5.5.1.1 Main features

For maximum versatility in the SmartCam configuration it has been implemented an extensible and editable modular structure (Figure 5.5). Furthermore, the SmartCam (see Figure 5.6) has been realized so as to ensure:

- Small size (40 × 40 mm) for easy installation in residential places.
- Low power consumption: it is equipped with an external battery and an intelligent power management system.
- A high-definition scanned images (up to 10 megapixel).
- Ability to communicate this information to the outside.
    1. **FORM OPTICAL:** the optical module includes a standard M12. A wide range of optics are commercially available.
    2. **SENSOR MODULE:** after appropriate analysis it was found that for the individual recognition a resolution of 5 megapixel is sufficient.
    3. **IMAGE ACQUISITION MODULE:** processes the images detected by the sensor and it is equipped with a flash memory to store the acquisitions.
    4. **MASTER MODULE:** it is the controller and the power supply of the other modules. It features low-power technology that allows a battery life of up to 6 months. It includes a microcontroller, non-volatile memory, a USB port,

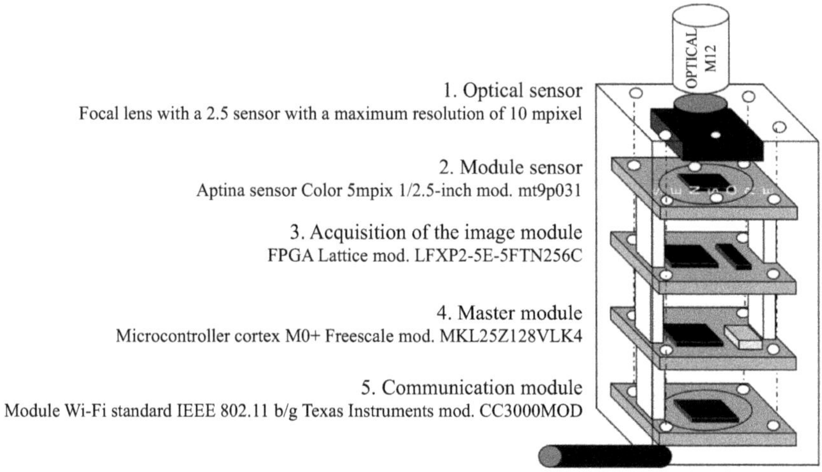

Figure 5.5 SmartCam modules

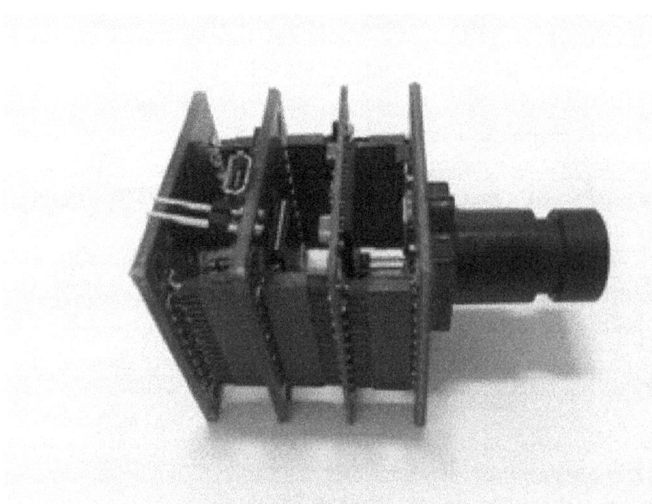

Figure 5.6 SmartCam prototype

connectors for connection with other modules, a battery input to 3.6 V and stabilizers necessary to organize other forms turn them off when not needed.

5. **COMMUNICATION MODULE:** a Wi-Fi data transmission module was added since most homes already have a wireless router that uses this standard. It provides the connectors for connection with the master module, the Wi-Fi radio module, the antenna and the stabilizer controlled by the master module.

5.5.2 SmartTv

Television is a device easily found in every home and is heavily used by people who have a sedentary lifestyle. Furthermore, it is one of the few who know how to use technological tools almost all older people, which generally have a technologies rejection. These reasons have led us to want to extend the capabilities of commercial television, by implementing a system that can monitor user activity weak during use and interact with him. The interaction with the elderly as well as provide important data to highlight the occurrence of any disturbances, has also allowed us to reduce the damaging effects of television, an instrument that leads to a pseudo sedation (reference article found) intellectual and a lack of social and emotional stimuli. The main features implemented are:

- The state of the SmartTv and reading of parameters of use (apps, channels, content, etc.).
- The activation of interactive systems and analytical applications.
- Reading in the background of test results or games aimed at collecting data on the habits.
- Sending messages and information to the user.

An analysis of the most widespread SmartTv commercial devices on the market was made to verify the possibility to implement the required functionality by the AngelHome project on these devices. They were taken into account some of the main reference manufacturers: Samsung, Sony, Panasonic, Toshiba, LG. It was verified the lack of standardization of the features and specifications of various brands. There is not the possibility to access from the outside with a protocol structured to information devices and present application. The considered manufacturers offer the opportunity to develop dedicated applications, but often there is not a standard in the programming language (html, Android) and made available in bookstores. A test to analyze the performance using a SmartTv Samsung H5500 (Screen 40 "Dual Core" 2.30 GHz processor, 2 GB of RAM, Android System 32-bit) has been carried out. In this device it has been installed a generic application for image processing and the following activities were measured: Extraction of edges using Canny algorithm [29], replacement of color pixels using pixel find and replace algorithms [30] and feature extraction point using Speeded Up Robust Feature (SURF) algorithm [31].

Five mega pixel images have been used in input, the performance of the device were compared with the performance of these algorithms on commercial Cubes Board based on ARM A9 with 2 GB of RAM and all three calculations, the average processing time of single frame are superior results for the SmartTv of 48 per cent on average highlighting the high exploitation that the part of drivers, and all the video streams management components have on internal hardware. This evidence has led the working group to consider the need to create a smart box dedicated to the vision and sensor technology and specialized in processing. For the implementation of the device interface was of paramount importance these search criteria by the BE THERE based on interviews carried out on older people because it allowed to have important information about their needs and preferences (see Figure 5.7).

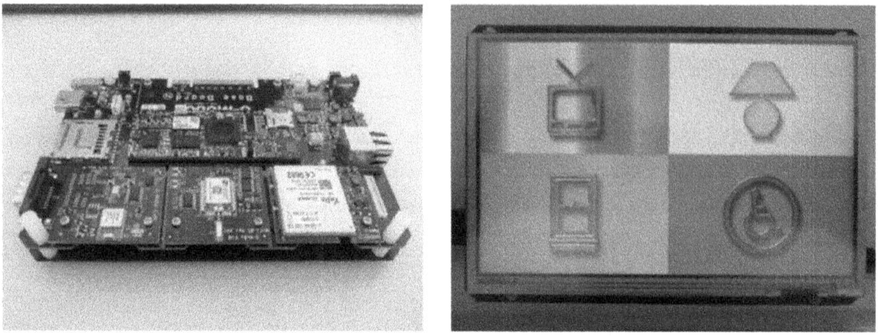

Figure 5.7 SmartTv prototype

5.6 Classification and machine learning

Taking into account the state of art, the first aspect that is clear is that the classification systems of behavior are heavily influenced by the subject: the emotions, reactions and the weak user behavior can be many and vary from person to person. This premise leads to the need to develop a classification system based on a model that must possess an adaptive character and self-calibrating on the subject under examination. Not only the overall psychological well-being but also the psychological and relational aspects of the user must be the core of the classification system so that the model must necessarily be user centered.

In AngelHome project was implemented a software that manages the emotions, reactions and behaviors of users, developed into a web server, which provides a machine learning module that is able to learn from the acquired data. The available data on AngelHome are: those collected from smart cameras allocated in different parts of the home environment, the data recorded by interaction with the SmartTv and data from sensors of comfort. The data resulting from the SmartCam have been studied through the template matching method [32] that allows, through the image reworking, to recognize the movements, the postures and the holding time in these positions the user. The software in this way can recognize the attitudes that the subject will show more frequently classifying these as typical behaviors. Very useful for the determination of "normal" behavior were interviews on cognitive psychological behaviors discussed previously. Reworking a classification of abnormal behavior may be programmed to automatically transmit alarm: the user, the family, or caregiver or emergency vehicles, where there was need.

5.6.1 Analyzing data in AngelHome: behavior and classification sensors

The main purpose was to be able to learn from proper processes and classify them, and then manage and detect any abnormal behavior that may be due to internal alarm situations to housing. This process of analysis will also allow to retrieve new information otherwise impossible to extrapolate (small changes in behavior would be difficult to detect even by an expert who monitors the elderly 24 hours; 24 also would have a very high cost). Data available in AngelHome are those related to smart sensors inside the home automation, specifically:

- SmartCam: able to recognize the patient's positions and attitudes that can be traced to a deterioration of the faculties psycho cognitive.
- SmartTv: can retrieve information on interactions with the device, so as to highlight abnormal behavior by the elderly.
- stores information from the various environmental sensors (thermometer, humidity, noise, etc.) in order to be able to learn and train the system which will then make decisions to maintain a state of adequate comfort. In case of harmful air quality can for example automatically open the windows or send alarms to the outside by calling or texting.

Now the classification system is designed to retrieve and store information in a database; to implement a system of rules and behaviors to which you will have to follow the decision-making system is required the contribution of experts in the various medical and social fields which define the pattern on which to train the system.

5.7 Conclusion and future works

The project AngelHome aims to design and develop an innovative home automation system for the analysis of physical behavior and the decay of the mental capacities of vulnerable users, built-in automatic and interactive control of the safety and comfort of the home and the person. The project was carried out by an aggregation of eight SMEs and two research institutes, and was financed by the Marche region. The project combines two main objectives: the first is to analyze the behavior of the elderly or disabled person inside the house by monitoring his movements and actions accomplished during the day. This was possible thanks to the development of appropriate smart objects, in particular a low-cost SmartCamera able to detect the presence and movements of subjects and thanks to a SmartTv with capabilities of monitoring the actions carried out (watched channels, schedules, etc.) and special interactive programs to maintain the mental faculties. The second objective is to analyze and provide comfort and environmental safety within the home. This has been made possible thanks to a series of smart sensors integrated among them and able to measure environmental values (temperature, humidity, CO_2, etc.). One of the main innovative aspects of the project is to integrate the two areas with an automatic learning system able to make decisions independently on the basis of the acquired knowledge. It was therefore implemented an automatic analysis system of psychic decay through weak user data from SmartTv and SmartCam and it was implemented an automated analysis system of comfort based on the tenant's behavior and habits in order to maintain a standard of consistent environmental comfort. The whole system is equipped with a network infrastructure capable of concentrating data from several houses and provides different interfaces to access the data. It also comes with an automatic alert generation system via phone call or SMS ensuring a high security.

Finally, the platform ensures a high interoperability, allowing to easily add new smart objects thanks to the use of standard protocols and numerous interface technologies. Regarding future developments, we want to improve SmartCam adding an infrared sensor that can monitor weak people even in the absence of light. It also wants to integrate a video analysis sensor inside the SmartTv capable of monitoring the emotions and states of mind of the user.

Acknowledgments

This research is part of important projects funded by Università Politecnica delle Marche with important regional companies: Angel Home, Smartbox e FIT. The authors would like to thank every company for their support and job.

References

[1] A. C. Enthoven, *Theory and Practice of Managed Competition in Health Care Finance*. North-Holland, Elsevier, 2014.
[2] C. W. Hansen, "Health and development: A neoclassical perspective," *Health*, vol. 7, no. 3, pp. 274–295, 2013.
[3] W. H. Organization. (2007) 10 facts on ageing and the life course. Accessed: 2015-01-30. [Online]. Available: www.who.int/features/factfiles/ageing/en/
[4] K. Giannakouris. (2008) Eurostat: Statistics in focus population and social conditions, Switzerland, 72/2008.
[5] S. Patel, H. Park, P. Bonato, L. Chan, and M. Rodgers, "A review of wearable sensors and systems with application in rehabilitation," *Journal of Neuroengineering and rehabilitation*, vol. 9, no. 1, p. 21, 2012.
[6] M. J. O'Grady, C. Muldoon, M. Dragone, R. Tynan, and G. M. O'Hare, "Towards evolutionary ambient assisted living systems," *Journal of Ambient Intelligence and Humanized Computing*, vol. 1, no. 1, pp. 15–29, 2010.
[7] E. Frontoni, A. Mancini, and P. Zingaretti, "RGB-D sensors for human activity detection in AAL environments," in *Ambient Assisted Living*. Switzerland, Springer, 2014, pp. 127–135.
[8] J. C. Augusto, H. Nakashima, and H. Aghajan, "Ambient intelligence and smart environments: A state of the art," in *Handbook of ambient intelligence and smart environments*. Switzerland, Springer, 2010, pp. 3–31.
[9] M. Contigiani, E. Frontoni, A. Mancini, and A. Gatto, "Indoor people localization and tracking using an energy harvesting smart floor," in *2014 IEEE/ASME 10th International Conference on Mechatronic and Embedded Systems and Applications (MESA)*. Italy, IEEE, 2014, pp. 1–5.
[10] D. Liciotti, G. Massi, E. Frontoni, A. Mancini, and P. Zingaretti, "Human activity analysis for in-home fall risk assessment," in *2015 IEEE International Conference on Communication Workshop (ICCW)*. London, UK, IEEE, 2015, pp. 284–289.

[11] M. Mubashir, L. Shao, and L. Seed, "A survey on fall detection: Principles and approaches," *Neurocomputing*, vol. 100, pp. 144–152, 2013.
[12] D. Liciotti, M. Contigiani, E. Frontoni, A. Mancini, P. Zingaretti, and V. Placidi, "Shopper analytics: A customer activity recognition system using a distributed RGB-D camera network," in *Video Analytics for Audience Measurement*. Switzerland, Springer, 2014, pp. 146–157.
[13] E. Frontoni, A. Mancini, P. Zingaretti, and V. Placidi, "Information management for intelligent retail environment: The shelf detector system," *Information*, vol. 5, no. 2, pp. 255–271, 2014.
[14] E. Frontoni, P. Raspa, A. Mancini, P. Zingaretti, and V. Placidi, "Customers' activity recognition in intelligent retail environments," in *New Trends in Image Analysis and Processing–ICIAP 2013*. Springer, 2013, pp. 509–516.
[15] E. Aarts and R. Wichert, *Ambient Intelligence*. Springer, 2009.
[16] P. Remagnino and G. L. Foresti, "Ambient intelligence: A new multidisciplinary paradigm," *IEEE Transactions on Systems, Man and Cybernetics, Part A: Systems and Humans*, vol. 35, no. 1, pp. 1–6, 2005.
[17] C. Ramos, J. C. Augusto, and D. Shapiro, "Ambient intelligence – the next step for artificial intelligence," *IEEE Intelligent Systems*, vol. 23, no. 2, pp. 15–18, 2008.
[18] K. Ducatel, M. Bogdanowicz, F. Scapolo, J. Leijten, and J.-C. Burgelman, *Scenarios for Ambient Intelligence in 2010*. Office for Official Publications of the European Communities, 2001.
[19] R. Casas, R. B. Marín, A. Robinet, *et al.*, *User Modelling in Ambient Intelligence for Elderly and Disabled People*. Switzerland, Springer, 2008.
[20] P. L. Emiliani and C. Stephanidis, "Universal access to ambient intelligence environments: Opportunities and challenges for people with disabilities," *IBM Systems Journal*, vol. 44, no. 3, pp. 605–619, 2005.
[21] T. Kleinberger, M. Becker, E. Ras, A. Holzinger, and P. Müller, "Ambient intelligence in assisted living: Enable elderly people to handle future interfaces," in *Universal Access in Human–Computer Interaction. Ambient Interaction*. Switzerland, Springer, 2007, pp. 103–112.
[22] L. Atzori, A. Iera, and G. Morabito, "The internet of things: A survey," *Computer Networks*, vol. 54, no. 15, pp. 2787–2805, 2010.
[23] A. Dohr, R. Modre-Opsrian, M. Drobics, D. Hayn, and G. Schreier, "The internet of things for ambient assisted living," in *2010 Seventh International Conference on Information Technology: New Generations (ITNG)*. Las Vegas, Nevada, IEEE, 2010, pp. 804–809.
[24] J. Gubbi, R. Buyya, S. Marusic, and M. Palaniswami, "Internet of Things (IoT): A vision, architectural elements, and future directions," *Future Generation Computer Systems*, vol. 29, no. 7, pp. 1645–1660, 2013.
[25] M. R. Alam, M. B. I. Reaz, and M. A. M. Ali, "A review of smart homes—past, present, and future," *IEEE Transactions on System, Man, Cybernetics C, Applied Reviews*, vol. 42, no. 6, pp. 1190–1203, 2012.
[26] L. Rossi, A. Belli, A. De Santis, *et al.*, "Interoperability issues among smart home technological frameworks," in *2014 IEEE/ASME 10th International*

Conference on Mechatronic and Embedded Systems and Applications (MESA). Senigallia, IEEE, 2014, pp. 1–7.

[27] P. Baldi and S. Brunak, *Bioinformatics: The Machine Learning Approach*. London, England, MIT Press, 2001.

[28] E. Frontoni, A. Mancini, and P. Zingaretti, "Embedded vision sensor network for planogram maintenance in retail environments," *Sensors*, vol. 15, no. 9, pp. 21 114–21 133, 2015.

[29] J. Canny, "A computational approach to edge detection," *IEEE Transactions on Pattern Analysis and Machine Intelligence*, vol. PAMI-8, no. 6, pp. 679–698, 1986.

[30] M. İlsever and C. Ünsalan, "Pixel-based change detection methods," in *Two-Dimensional Change Detection Methods*. Switzerland, Springer, 2012, pp. 7–21.

[31] H. Bay, A. Ess, T. Tuytelaars, and L. Van Gool, "Speeded-up robust features (SURF)," *Computer Vision and Image Understanding*, vol. 110, no. 3, pp. 346–359, 2008.

[32] R. Brunelli, *Front Matter*. Wiley Online Library, 2009.

Chapter 6
Multi-sensor platform for circadian rhythm analysis

Pietro Siciliano, Alessandro Leone, Andrea Caroppo, Giovanni Diraco, and Gabriele Rescio

Abstract

Irregular patterns in the circadian rhythm may cause health problems, such as psychological or neurological disorders. Consequently, early detection of anomalies in circadian rhythm could be useful for the prevention of such problems. This work describes a multi-sensor platform for anomalies detection in circadian rhythm. The inputs of the platform are sequences of human postures, extensively used for analysis of activities of daily living and, more in general, for human behaviour understanding. The postures are acquired by using both ambient and wearable sensors that are time-of-flight 3D vision sensor, ultra-wideband radar sensor and triaxial accelerometer. The suggested platform aims to provide an abstraction layer with respect to the underlying sensing technologies, exploiting the postural information in common to all involved sensors (i.e., standing, bending, sitting, lying down). Furthermore, in order to fill the lack of datasets containing long-term postural sequences, which are required in circadian rhythm analysis, a simulator of activities of daily living/postures has been proposed. The capability of the platform in providing a sensing invariant interface (i.e., abstracted from any specific sensing technology) was demonstrated by preliminary results, exhibiting high accuracy in circadian rhythm anomalies detection using the three aforementioned sensors.

6.1 Introduction

The demography distribution of the developed world is set to change dramatically over the coming decades. Current trends show that the elderly population is increasing in size and this phenomenon is predicted to continue in the future. More specifically, in 2010, an estimated 524 million people were aged 65 or older (8% of the world's population). By 2050, this number is expected to nearly triple to about 1.5 billion, representing 16% of the world's population [1,2]. This trend of population ageing is as a result of reduction in fertility combined with increase in life expectancy. The increase in life expectancy is a positive situation, but there are a number of related effects that require consideration, such as the growth of the cognitive and physical impairment rate due to the ageing. As the effects of such an illness requires constant assistance, coupled with the financial infeasibility and limited number of care institutions; in this context, the need to explore new solutions is considered essential. Indeed it has been demonstrated that the institutionalisation and hospitalisation are considered as highly unfavourable consequences because as the majority of individuals prefer to remain at home [3].

Therefore, two related priorities in research are presented by the novel and effective methods for activity levels assessment at home and for the long-term monitoring and management of chronic conditions with the purpose of alleviating the increased strain on healthcare resources. The use of sensing technology within Intelligent Environments (IEs) is one such approach which has the potential to facilitate these needs [4]. IEs can provide objective data describing behaviour and health status allowing the development of reliable, privacy–preserving and automatic solutions for activity recognition, assisted living or healthcare monitoring. In this way it is possible to reduce the need of assistance from medical staff or caregiver for elderlies, favouring their healthy and independent life at home.

Smart sensors are becoming more and more a technology key in Ambient Assisted Living (AAL) scenarios. By focusing on the users' lifestyle, advancement in sensor technologies give us the opportunity to recognise Activities of Daily Living (ADLs) [5] for a long-period of time. Continuous monitoring of ADLs is helpful for detection of lifestyle disorders. Irregular patterns in the sleep/wake cycle, for example, may cause health problems, such as disorders of psychological or neurological nature. Consequently, early detection of abnormalities in the Circadian Rhythm (CR) can be useful for the prevention of such problems. In literature many approaches have been proposed for behaviour monitoring, reporting information about user's health and life patterns [6,7]. On the other hand, in [8–10] some methodologies for the detection of abnormal behaviour patterns are described. In the above systems, features obtained from a single sensing technology are considered (e.g., pressure sensor, motion sensor, presence infrared sensor, wearable sensor). In these works, using probabilistic approaches, detection and classification of abnormal behaviour patterns are reached with a good level of accuracy. However, these systems have some limitations. In fact, they have no ability to manage long-term data and in some circumstances a training phase is required.

This paper reports the description of a multi-sensor platform for detection of anomalies in human sleep patterns within AAL context by using an unsupervised methodology. The input of the system is constituted by sequences of human postures generated by using an activity simulation approach specifically designed and implemented within this work. The use of postures is motivated by their extensive use in ADLs modelling [11], besides that ADL sequences allow to model human behaviour.

The rest of the paper is organised as follows. Section 6.2 reports, for each sensing approach, the computational frameworks for posture detection (detection layer). Moreover, in the same section, the general architecture of the data simulation tool is described, providing some information about the methodology used for simulation of ADLs and generation of long-term postures (simulation layer). Finally, in the last subsection, the feature extraction procedure and the unsupervised classification of CR anomalies is detailed (reasoning layer). The experimental results are reported in Section 6.3 and discussed in Section 6.4. Finally, conclusive considerations are provided in Section 6.5.

6.2 Materials and methods

The multi-sensor platform software architecture is organised, as shown in Figure 6.1, in three main layers: detection layer, simulation layer and reasoning layer.

The detection layer provides sequences of human postures detected by three different sensors: a Time-Of-Flight (TOF) sensor, a Ultra-wideband (UWB) radar and an ST MEMS triaxial accelerometer (ACC). The first two (TOF, UWB) approaches refer to ambient solutions, whereas the last one falls into wearable ones.

In the simulation layer, long-term posture sequences are generated according to a calibrated simulation, based on real-life experiments and conducted with the three aforementioned sensors.

The reasoning layer offers an automatic tool for the detection of anomalies in CR by using an unsupervised methodology. It is important to highlight the platform capability in providing a technology invariant interface abstract from any specific sensing technology.

6.2.1 Detection layer

Human postures can be detected by using posture detection approaches that are differently characterised in terms of invasiveness, accuracy, robustness to object occlusion and cluttering, and data richness, as summarised in Table 6.1.

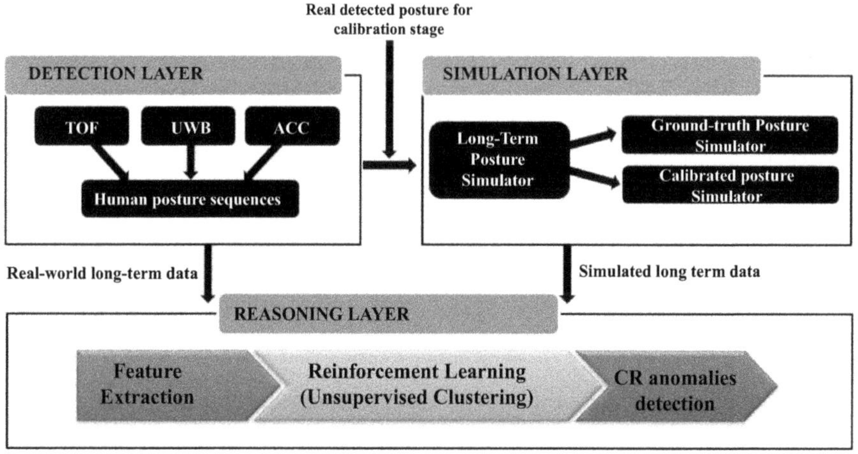

Figure 6.1 Implemented logic modules overview

Table 6.1 *Comparison of three posture detectors*

Characteristic	TOF	UWB	ACC
Invasiveness	Low	Very low	Medium
Accuracy	Very high	Medium	Medium
Robustness to object occlusion and cluttering	Low	High	Very high
Data richness	Very high	Medium	Medium

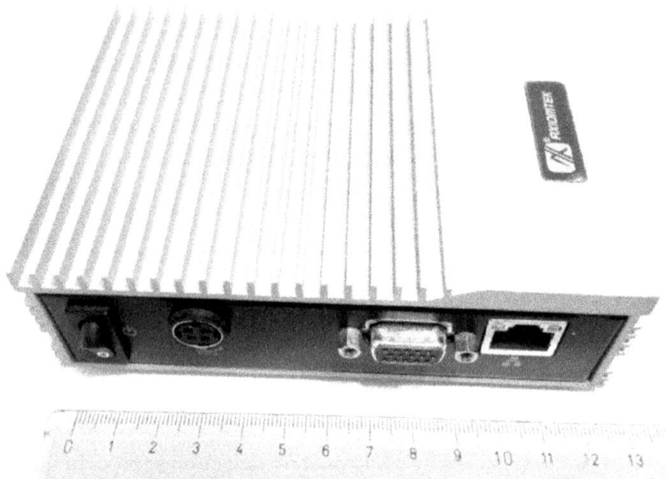

Figure 6.2 *Embedded-PC running detection algorithms*

Each posture detector provides as output a sequence of postures, with variable detail levels (i.e., data richness) depending on the sensing approach used. As already mentioned, four postures have been taken into account in this study: Standing (St), Bending (Be), Sitting (Si), and Lying down (Ly), although certain approaches (e.g., vision-based) are able to recognise a far greater number of postures. For all approaches, the detection algorithms ran on the fan-less embedded-PC equipped with Intel® Atom™ processor shown in Figure 6.2. The following subsections describe each detection approach in detail.

6.2.1.1 TOF-based posture detector

This detector adopts the MESA SR-4000 [12] shown in Figure 6.3, a state-of-the-art TOF sensor having compact (65 × 65 × 68 mm) dimensions, noiseless (0 dB) working, QCIF (176 × 144 pixels) resolution, long (10 m) distance range, wide (69° × 56°) field-of-view, and low power (9.6 W) consumption. The TOF-based posture recognition is inspired by the work of Diraco *et al.* [13]. At early processing level, the

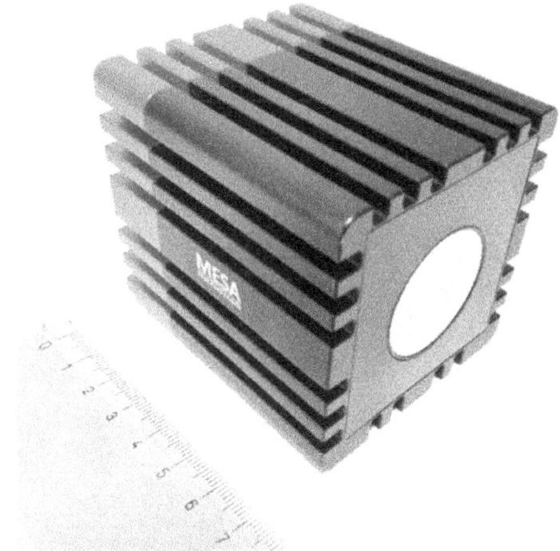

Figure 6.3 MESA SR-4000 TOF sensor

computational framework includes a self-calibration procedure to allow for easy installation of the TOF sensor, without requiring neither calibration objects nor user intervention. The self-calibration makes use of the popular RANSAC-based plane detector to identify the position of the floor, which is used to estimate the extrinsic calibration parameters. Moving foreground objects are extracted from calibrated range data by modelling the background with a mixture of Gaussian and segmenting the foreground with a Bayesian classifier. Finally, people are detected and tracked using the CONDENSATION (Conditional Density Propagation) algorithm. The remaining part of the computational framework focuses on feature extraction and posture classification. The intrinsic topology of a generic shape, i.e. a human body scan captured via TOF sensor, is graphically encoded by using the concept of Discrete Reeb Graph (DRG) proposed by Xiao *et al.* [14]. To extract the DRG, the Geodesic distance is used as invariant Morse function [15] since it is invariant not only to translation, scale and rotation but also to isometric transformations ensuring high accuracy in body parts representation under postural changes. The geodesic distance map is computed by using a two-step procedure. Firstly, a connected mesh, shown in Figure 6.4(a), is built on the 3D point cloud by using the nearest-neighbour rule. Secondly, given a starting point M (i.e. the body's centroid) the geodesic distance between M and each other mesh node is computed as the shortest path on mesh by using an efficient implementation of Dijkstra's algorithm suggested by Verroust and Lazarus [16]. The computed geodesic map is shown in Figure 6.4(b) in which grey levels represent geodesic distances.

The DRG is extracted by subdividing the geodesic map in regular level-sets and connecting them on the basis of an adjacency criterion as described by Diraco *et al.* [13] that suggests also a methodology to handle self-occlusions (due to overlapping body parts). The DRG-based features are shown in Figure 6.4(c) and represented by the

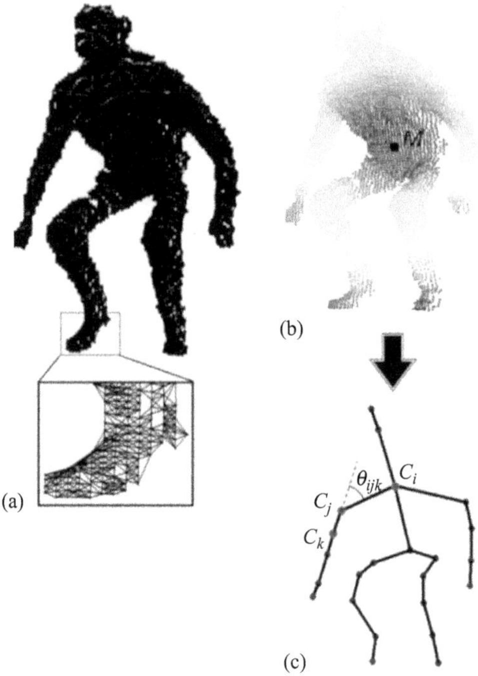

Figure 6.4 TOF-based features: (a) mesh, (b) geodesic map, and (c) DRG-based features

topological descriptor that includes DRG nodes {Ci,Cj,Ck} and related angles {ϑijk}. A multiclass formulation of the Support Vector Machine (SVM) classifier [17] based on the one-against-one strategy is adopted to classify (St, Be, Si, Ly) postures. Since interesting results have been reported with the Radial Basis Function (RBF) kernel for posture recognition [18], such a kernel is used and associated parameters, namely regularisation constant K and the kernel argument γ, are tuned according to a global grid search strategy.

6.2.1.2 UWV-based posture detector

This detector adopts the PulsON 410 manufactured by Time Domain Corporation [19] shown in Figure 6.5, a state-of-the-art UWB radar sensor, having a good wall penetration capability (2 GHz bandwidth), RF transmissions from 3.1 GHz to 5.3 GHz centred at 4.3 GHz, compact (76 $\times$ 80 $\times$ 16 mm) board dimensions, and it is able to operate in both mono- and multi-static configurations. UWB radar sensors find many applications ranging from vital signs detection to target localisation and tracking, not only in contactless modality but also through the walls. In this study, the PulsON 410 sensor is used for recognition of human postures regardless to the presence of large occluding objects (e.g., pieces of furniture, walls) interposed between target and sensor.

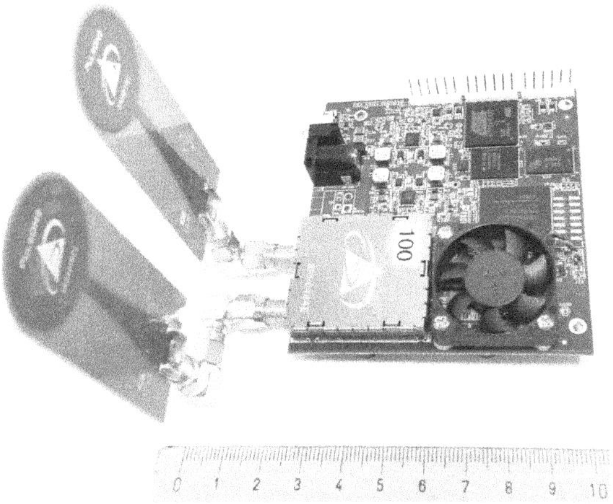

Figure 6.5 The PulsON 410 UWB radar in monostatic setup

The computational framework includes three main stages: (1) the pre-processing for clutter reduction/removal, (2) the feature extraction, and (3) the posture classification. At the pre-processing stage, after band-pass filtering (Butterworth IIR 16th order) with a transition band of 3.1–5.3 GHz for filtering out frequencies outside the transmitter range, the clutter is removed by using the Running Gaussian Average technique for background subtraction [20]. In Figure 6.6 some examples of the filtered signals for the lying down and the sitting postures are reported. Given the Time-Of-Arrival (TOA) corresponding to the component of the human body, the feature extraction stage is based on the estimation of the following quantities: normalised energy, variance, skewness, kurtosis, as defined in [21]. Finally, the feature vector is classified by means of ensemble classification technique based on Real AdaBoost [22]. The AdaBoost classifier was trained by using the 10% of posture sequences, instead the remaining sequences were used for testing.

6.2.1.3 ACC-based posture detector

The wearable device used in this version of the platform is the Wearable Wellness System (WWS), produced by Smartex [23]. It made up of a sensorised garment and an electronic device (SEW) for the acquisition, the storage and the wireless transmission of the data. It has been designed to continuously monitor main vital parameters (ECG, Heart rate, Breathe rate) and the movements. The WWS garment is suitable and comfortable, reducing the well-known usability problems of the smart wearable devices. Moreover it can be washed and it can be in tight contact with the body without any creases. In Figure 6.7 the male version of the t-shirt is shown.

It integrates (a) two textile electrodes, (b) one textile piezoresistive sensor and (c) a pocket, placed on the chest, for the SEW electronic device in which it is integrated a triaxial MEMS accelerometer for the movement monitoring. The WWS can operate

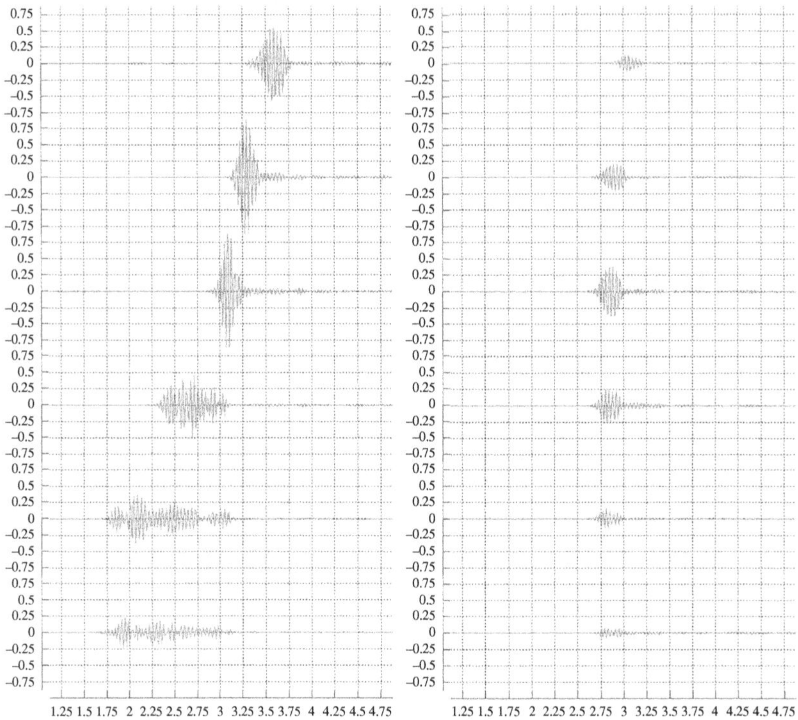

Figure 6.6 Filtered radar scans for two different postures: lying down on the bed (left) and sitting on the chair (right)

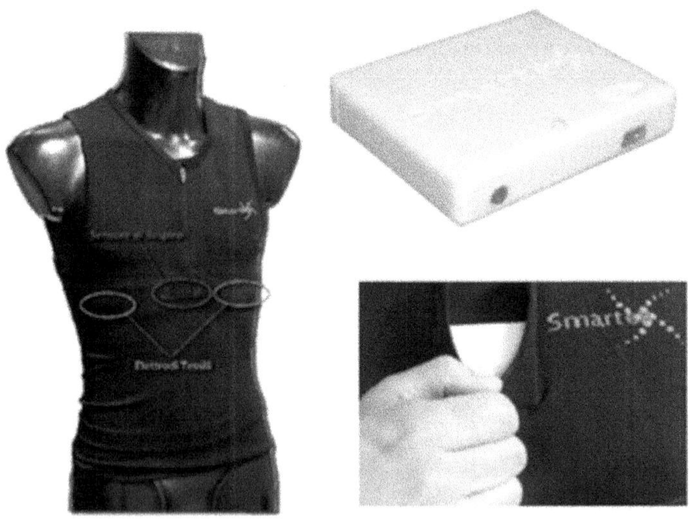

Figure 6.7 Smartex Wearable Wellness System

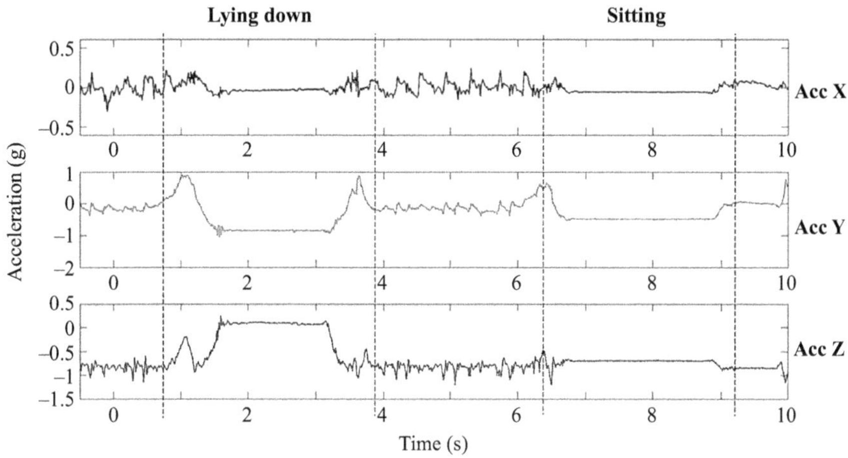

Figure 6.8 Example of acceleration data along the three axes for the classification of two different postures (lying down and sitting)

in streaming, via Bluetooth up to 20 meters (in free space), or in off-line modality, storing the data on a micro-SD integrated in the SEW device. In streaming mode the duration of its rechargeable battery life is about 8 hours, while in off-line the duration is more than 18 hours. For the elaboration, the raw acceleration data have been sent to the embedded PC with a 25 Hz frequency, that it is enough to recognise the physical activity [24]. The data are in the decimal format and represent the acceleration values with full scale in the range of ±2g and a 10 bit resolution for an high sensitivity. The MEMS accelerometer is DC coupled, so it measures both static and dynamic acceleration along the three axes and allows to get information on the 3D spatial relative position (compared to the Earth gravity vector) of the person who wears it. Indeed, if the accelerometer relative orientation is known, the resulting data can be used to determinate the angle α of the user position with respect to the vertical direction. In Figure 6.8 some examples of the raw acceleration data along the three axes for the lying down and the sitting postures are shown. The main computational steps of the software architecture for the posture recognition are: data acquisition, data pre-processing, system calibration, feature extraction and classification. Data are converted into gravitational unit to represent acceleration data in the range of ±2g, in order to make possible to extract the angle α and avoiding different orders of magnitude in the features. The samples coming from the device are filtered out by a low-pass FIR filter to reduce the noise due to the electronic components, environment and human tremor. In order to correctly handle the pre-processed data, a calibration procedure was accomplished by recovering the initial conditions after the device mounting. The features extracted to detect the posture are: the Averaged Acceleration Energy (AAE), the mean and the standard deviation [25] over three acceleration axes by using a 5 s sliding window. Moreover the features obtained in [26] are used; they consider the variation of dynamic acceleration and the change of position during a sitting/lying/standing up actions with respect to an upright position. The classification of the (St, Be, Si, Ly) postures is obtained by implementing the effective and robust semi-supervised k-means clustering algorithm and Euclidean distance [27].

6.2.2 Simulation layer

Since the availability of datasets for behaviour analysis is limited by difficulties in the collection of such data, and considered the lack of datasets containing long-term postural sequences, a simulator of ADLs/postures has been implemented within this work. The simulator provides virtual data with the ability to rapidly generate a large simulated dataset driven by different parameters, which allow to reproduce different normal/anomalous behaviours (referred in particular to CR patterns).

The simulator is made up of two stages, one for simulation of long-term ADLs and another one for simulation of long-term postures referred to a specific sensing approach.

6.2.2.1 Long-term ADLs simulator

The general architecture of the simulator is inspired from the work of Noury *et al.* [28]. The authors assumed that the daily activities of a subject are almost regular. Thus, the simulator is based on a Markov model with homogeneous periods, while the time for transitions is ruled by a Finite State Machine (FSM) [29]. The Markov chains are frequently used to represent a Bayesian process with multiple states and their associated conditional probabilities. Thus the use of HMM seems a suitable probabilistic approach to model the whole system.

As shown in Figure 6.9, the day is segmented into seven periods (e.g., wake up, morning, lunch, afternoon, dinner, going to bed, sleep) and thus seven Markov models corresponding to well-identified circadian rhythms were modelled. In this way, each period can be represented by a graph of the transitions (used for the translation in activity sequences that can occur during the specific daily period) that are controlled by their probabilities. The simulated data are structured in the following matrix expression: $M = $ [Date, StartTime, EndTime, Activity], where Date, StartTime, EndTime and Activity are column vector representing respectively the date of the simulation day (expressed in the following format: dd/mm/yyyy), the start time and the end time of the simulated activity (expressed in the following format: hh:mm:ss) and the name of the latter.

Each period of the day is modelled using an N-states HMM in which N represents the ADLs performed during the period itself. As an example, the three states HMM modelling the "morning" period is reported in Figure 6.10. The next step of the simulator is devoted to translate activities in a sequence of actions. In this work, an action is an atomic element which provides the details of a specific activity. For example, the activity "have breakfast" is translated by the following sequence of actions: "prepare breakfast" – "breakfast" – "washing up".

The assumption made in this version of the simulator is always to translate each activity with the same sequence of actions, only varying the time duration.

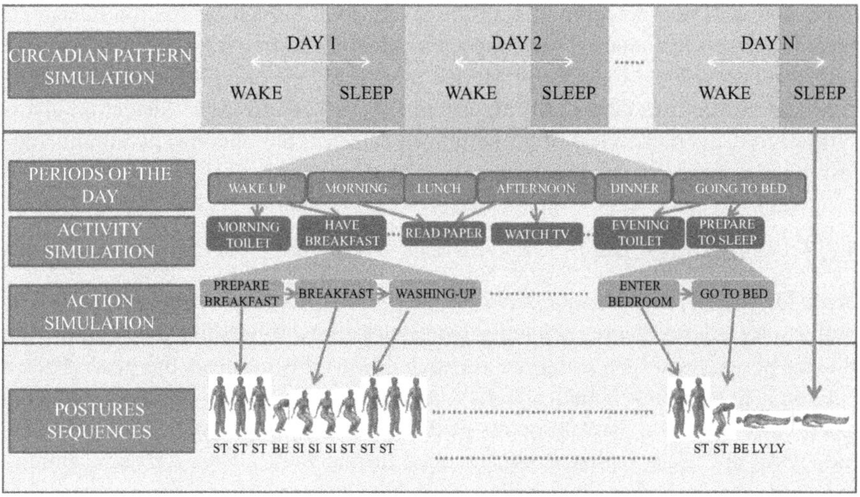

Figure 6.9 Conceptual representation of the posture simulator (SI = Sitting, ST = Standing, BE = Bending, LY = Lying Down)

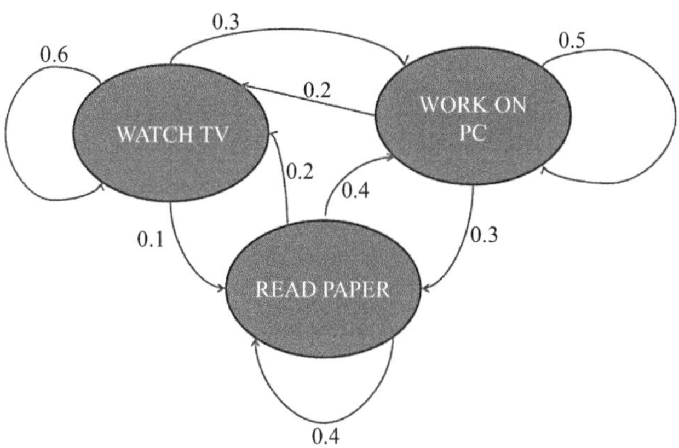

Figure 6.10 Markov model for the representation of the period of the day "morning" with three states

Finally, as described in the next subsection, the last layer of the simulator is addressed to model each action as a sequence of the postures (taking into account the only four postures previously mentioned).

6.2.2.2 Long-term posture simulator

Starting from the sequence of actions provided by the ADLs simulator, the posture sequence is generated by using a calibrated approach based on real observations conducted with real detectors (i.e., TOF, UWB, ACC). Such calibration consists in modelling errors introduced by each specific detector, starting from simulated ground-truth sequences. The Model Error Modelling (MEM) method [30] together with the Expectation-Maximisation (EM) algorithm [31] is used to model detection errors. Furthermore, the parameters of the simulated detectors are obtained by minimising a cost function based on the Prediction Error Method (PEM) [32].

6.2.3 Reasoning layer

Given long-term posture sequences referred to the different sensing approaches, the platform includes a feature extraction procedure aimed to identify the starting point of sleep periods and their durations for each day. At this purpose, the most efficient solution is to recognise human actions from patterns of posture sequences, and more specifically to extract starting points of the actions: "going to bed", "sleep in bed" and "wake up". The approach implemented in this work allows ADLs recognition using the approach described below. Basically, human actions are recognised by considering successive postures over time periods. A transition action occurs when the person changes the current action to another action. Thus, a transition action might include several transition postures. Transition actions are merged together to form single atomic actions and global events are recognised by using Dynamic Bayesian Networks (DBNs) specifically designed for indoor application scenario, following an approach similar to Park and Kautz [33]. Designed DBNs have a hierarchical structure with three node layers: activity, interaction and sensor. The activity layer stays on top of hierarchy and includes hidden nodes to model high-level activities (i.e. ADLs, behaviours, etc.). The interaction layer is a hidden layer as well and it is devoted to model the states of evidence for interactions inside the home (i.e. appliances, furniture, locations, etc.). The detector layer, at the bottom of hierarchy, gathers data from detector sensors (postures). Each DBN is hence decomposed in multiple Hidden Markov Models (HMMs) including interaction and sensor layers, and trained on the basis of the Viterbi algorithm [34]. In this way, the detection of sleep start time can be derived from the recognition of the action "going to bed", and the duration of sleep can be obtained evaluating the difference between "wake up" time and "sleep in bed" time.

The aforementioned features (starting point of sleep and the relative duration extracted for each simulated day) are mapped in 2D space, in which the x-axis represents the start time of the sleep and the y-axis represents the relative time duration. Through the use of this representation, a normal CR generates a cluster which is composed of neighbouring points (that can be assumed as reference CR).

Subsequently, the algorithmic steps on the recording of any changes in the circadian rhythm are addressed through the use of a reinforcement learning procedure. The procedure is based on using an incremental clustering technique [35] that provides with an unsupervised approach a real-time discovery of changes in CR with respect to a reference CR. This is achieved by incrementally clustering incoming extracted features. In the simulator, different time intervals have been taken into account as reference period (labelled with M), followed by periods within which a change in the CR pattern was simulated (labelled with N). When a new cluster appears, a CR change is detected if the features belonging to the new cluster are extracted from N consecutive days (not necessary adjacent), with N set according to physician's indications.

6.3 Experimental results

In the current section, the results obtained in correspondence of each platform layer, described in Section 6.2, are reported.

The posture detection performance of each detector has been estimated by using a common experimental setup in which 18 healthy subjects (nine males and nine females, age 38 ± 6 years, height 175 ± 20 cm, weight 75 ± 22 kg) have been involved. The participants were asked to perform typical ADLs, such as household tasks, meal preparation, feeding, sitting and watching TV, relaxing and sleeping. During such experimental sessions, data were collected simultaneously by ambient-installed TOF and UWB, and an ACC worn by each participant. For each detector, the classification performance and the related averaged confusion matrix is provided in Table 6.2.

The feature extraction step has been evaluated on a series of experiments in which synthetic data were affected by different percentages of errors related to: (1) sensor noise and (2) fault situation which can occur in real contexts (e.g. wearable sensor not worn, vision sensor turned off or occluded, resulting in postures not available during

Table 6.2 Confusion matrices for TOF, UWB and ACC detector

TOF		**Predicted posture (%)**			
		St	**Be**	**Si**	**Ly**
Actual postures (%)	**St**	**99**	1	0	0
	Be	0	**97**	3	0
	Si	3	0	**97**	0
	Ly	0	2	0	**98**
UWB		**St**	**Be**	**Si**	**Ly**
Actual postures (%)	**St**	**82**	13	5	0
	Be	18	**75**	6	1
	Si	11	8	**79**	2
	Ly	0	4	15	**81**
ACC		**St**	**Be**	**Si**	**Ly**
Actual postures (%)	**St**	**92**	2	6	0
	Be	2	**84**	2	12
	Si	11	2	**87**	0
	Ly	0	5	1	**94**

Confusion matrices for TOF, UWB and ACC detector. The recognition rate for each posture class is highlighted in bold.

a time period). The purpose to simulate situations close to reality has been reached by modelling the noise with two kinds of components: bias noise (uniform distribution) and posture transition noise (Gaussian distribution). Performances have been evaluated in terms of Mean Absolute Error (MAE) by measuring the misalignment between ground-truth sleep phases (generated for each simulated day) and detected ones, and also in terms of Mean Relative Error (MRE) related to the percentage of undetected sleep phases. The previous error measurements are estimated through 10 synthetic datasets constituted by different time periods; the number of simulated days

Table 6.3 Evaluation of feature extraction step in terms of mean absolute error (MAE) and mean relative error (MRE)

Exp. #	**Days #**	**Bias noise %**	**Posture transition noise %**	**Fault situation %**	**Alignment MAE (minutes)**	**Detection MRE %**
1	120	0	0	0	**5**	**0**
2	90	20	10	0	**5.2**	**0**
3	150	20	30	0	**5.3**	**0**
4	90	30	10	0	**5.2**	**0**
5	90	30	30	0	**20.1**	**5**
6	120	20	10	15	**8.4**	**4**
7	120	20	30	15	**9.5**	**6**
8	90	30	10	15	**11.7**	**7**
9	150	20	10	30	**14.4**	**10**
10	120	30	30	30	**36.5**	**21**

The values reported in the column "Alignment MAE (in minutes)" correspond to the mean absolute error expressed in minutes and obtained measuring during each experiment the misalignment between the start time of ground-truth sleep phases and the detected ones for each simulated day. The values reported in the column "Detection MRE" correspond to the Mean Relative Error (expressed in %) of undetected sleep phases.

Table 6.4 Detection rate (%) of deviations from the reference CR at varying of M and N

***M* (days)**	**Detector**	***N* (days)**						
		7	**14**	**21**	**28**	**35**	**42**	**49**
60	**TOF**	76.4	**90.2**	90.7	94.6	95	95.8	96.5
	ACC	73.1	**84.6**	86.1	89.5	92.3	93.1	94.5
	UWB	69.7	73.5	77.2	**81.4**	84.5	87.7	90.2
120	**TOF**	72.1	74.4	**80.3**	88.7	88.9	89.2	90.5
	ACC	69.8	70.1	73.9	76.8	**80.2**	83.6	86.7
	UWB	65.2	67.6	70.2	73.5	78.5	**81.4**	82.9
180	**TOF**	60.4	73.7	79.7	**80.2**	87.4	88.9	90.4
	ACC	58.7	62.6	66.9	70.4	74.2	**79.7**	83.7
	UWB	56.4	60.1	63	67.9	72.7	77.5	**80**

Detection rate (%) of deviations from the reference CR at varying of M and N. The values in bold are referred to the numbers of days N that are at least necessary to obtain a minimum detection rate of 80% at varying of the reference period M.

for each experiment, the percentage of errors and relative performances are reported in Table 6.3.

For the validation of the incremental clustering step, a series of experiments that simulate three different reference periods (with a duration of M days) have been carried out. After each period, a change in CR pattern was simulated (with a duration of N days). The change was obtained perturbing randomly the sleep start time or its temporal duration. In Table 6.4, the detection rate of trend changes, at varying of both M and N, is reported for each detector:

6.4 Discussion

From the analysis of the obtained results, it is evident the platform ability and its high level of accuracy in identification of changes in CR. At the increasing of reference period, the incremental clustering achieves good performance if changes in CR pattern persist for a time period of greater duration. However, the performances are strictly related to the sensing technology involved; in fact, at varying of the detector, a different number of days N is required to reach a satisfactory detection rate. For example, if we consider a reference period of length $M = 120$ days, a detection rate of about 80% is reached within $N = 21$ days (TOF), $N = 35$ days (ACC), $N = 42$ days (UWB).

The platform has been validated by using posture sequences simulated in a calibrated way (with calibration error less than 2%) and referring to common ADLs carried out by older people in their home environment. Furthermore, the solution was tested considering reference periods M very different in order to taking into account any deviations with respect to standard execution of ADLs. This leads up to believe that the performances that can be reached using real monitoring systems should be included between $M = 60$ and $M = 180$, with N corresponding to the sensing technology used.

From a usability perspective, the platform is consistent with the independent living context, in fact the detection of changes in CR can be automatically obtained allowing offline analysis by a caregiver/doctor for subsequent clinical evaluations. It is important to stress the versatility of the platform: it can potentially operate with any kind of detector able to provide postural information. In particular, the platform has been validated by three detectors based on sensing principles that are all compatible with AAL scenario.

The added values of the multi-sensory platform described in this paper are easy to identify. First of all, the use of features such as the human postures enables the integration of multi-sensor devices which can reproduce the same set of features. Moreover, the functionality of the whole system could be extended acquiring as input different sets of features (e.g. motion level or spatial position) with the purpose to manage other disorders, such as sedentary or hyperkinetic behaviour.

6.5 Conclusion

The purpose of the present work was to design and evaluate a multi-sensor platform for detection of CR anomalies. The most significant contribution lies in the use of abstract features (human postures) produced by a generic detector, making the presented framework independent from a specific sensing technology. The suggested computational framework was optimised and validated for embedded processing in order to meet typical in-home application requirements such as low power consumption, noiselessness and compactness.

Three computational framework that include common main stages are designed and implemented in order to detect four human postures with both ambient and wearable sensing device. Moreover, the long-term data unavailability has been solved through the use of a simulator of ADLs/posture able to mimic the real behaviour of the sensors used in this work thanks to a calibrated approach.

Acknowledgements

This work was carried out within the project "ACTIVE AGEING AT HOME" funded by the Italian Ministry of Education, Universities and Research, within the National Operational Programme for "Research and Competitiveness" 2007–2013.

References

[1] "United nations department of economic and social affairs," (http://www.un.org/en/development/desa/population/), last access July 21, 2016.

[2] U. N. P. on Ageing, "The Ageing of the World's Population," (http://www.un.org/en/development/desa/population/publications/pdf/ageing/WorldPopulationAgeing2013.pdf), last access July 21, 2016.

[3] M. R. Gillick, N. A. Serrell, and L. S. Gillick, "Adverse consequences of hospitalization in the elderly," *Social Science & Medicine*, vol. 16, no. 10, pp. 1033–1038, 1982.

[4] L. Chen, C. D. Nugent, J. Biswas, and J. Hoey, *Activity Recognition in Pervasive Intelligent Environments*. Paris, France, Springer Science & Business Media, 2011, vol. 4.

[5] D. Barer and F. Nouri, "Measurement of activities of daily living," *Clinical Rehabilitation*, vol. 3, no. 3, pp. 179–187, 1989.

[6] G. Virone, M. Alwan, S. Dalal, *et al.*, "Behavioral patterns of older adults in assisted living," *IEEE Transactions on Information Technology in Biomedicine*, vol. 12, no. 3, pp. 387–398, 2008.

[7] A. A. Chaaraoui, J. R. Padilla-López, F. J. Ferrández-Pastor, M. Nieto-Hidalgo, and F. Flórez-Revuelta, "A vision-based system for intelligent monitoring: human behaviour analysis and privacy by context," *Sensors*, vol. 14, no. 5, pp. 8895–8925, 2014.

[8] G. Virone, N. Noury, and J. Demongeot, "A system for automatic measurement of circadian activity deviations in telemedicine," *IEEE Transactions on Biomedical Engineering*, vol. 49, no. 12, pp. 1463–1469, 2002.

[9] F. Cardinaux, S. Brownsell, M. Hawley, and D. Bradley, "Modelling of behavioural patterns for abnormality detection in the context of lifestyle reassurance," in *Iberoamerican Congress on Pattern Recognition*. Havana, Cuba, Springer, 2008, pp. 243–251.

[10] J. H. Shin, B. Lee, and K. S. Park, "Detection of abnormal living patterns for elderly living alone using support vector data description," *IEEE Transactions on Information Technology in Biomedicine*, vol. 15, no. 3, pp. 438–448, 2011.

[11] V. Kellokumpu, M. Pietikäinen, and J. Heikkilä, "Human activity recognition using sequences of postures." in *MVA*, 2005, pp. 570–573.

[12] "MESA Imaging AG, SR4000/SR4500 User Manual, Version 3.0," (http://www.realtechsupport.org/UB/SR/range_finding/SR4000_SR4500_Manual.pdf), last access July 21, 2016.

[13] G. Diraco, A. Leone, and P. Siciliano, "In-home hierarchical posture classification with a time-of-flight 3D sensor," *Gait & Posture*, vol. 39, no. 1, pp. 182–187, 2014.

[14] Y. Xiao, P. Siebert, and N. Werghi, "Topological segmentation of discrete human body shapes in various postures based on geodesic distance," in *Proceedings of the 17th International Conference on Pattern Recognition*, vol. 3. Cambridge, UK, IEEE, Aug. 2004, pp. 131–135.

[15] S. Baloch, H. Krim, I. Kogan, and D. Zenkov, "Rotation invariant topology coding of 2D and 3D objects using Morse theory," in *IEEE International Conference on Image Processing*, vol. 3. Genoa, Italy, IEEE, Sept. 2006, pp. III–796.

[16] A. Verroust and F. Lazarus, "Extracting skeletal curves from 3D scattered data," *The Visual Computer*, vol. 16, no. 1, pp. 15–25, 2000.

[17] R. Debnath, N. Takahide, and H. Takahashi, "A decision based one-against-one method for multi-class support vector machine," *Pattern Analysis and Applications*, vol. 7, no. 2, pp. 164–175, 2004.

[18] F. Buccolieri, C. Distante, and A. Leone, "Human posture recognition using active contours and radial basis function neural network," in *IEEE Conference on Advanced Video and Signal Based Surveillance*. Como, Italy, IEEE, Sept. 2005, pp. 213–218.

[19] "TIME DOMAIN, PulsON®410, P410 radar kit," (http://www.timedomain.com/p400-mrm.php), last access July 21, 2016.

[20] C. R. Wren, A. Azarbayejani, T. Darrell, and A. P. Pentland, "Pfinder: Real-time tracking of the human body," *IEEE Transactions on Pattern Analysis and Machine Intelligence*, vol. 19, no. 7, pp. 780–785, 1997.

[21] M. A. Kiasari, S. Y. Na, and J. Y. Kim, "Classification of human postures using ultra-wide band radar based on neural networks," in *International Conference on IT Convergence and Security (ICITCS)*. Beijing, China, IEEE, Oct. 2014, pp. 1–4.

[22] R. E. Schapire and Y. Singer, "Improved boosting algorithms using confidence-rated predictions," *Machine Learning*, vol. 37, no. 3, pp. 297–336, 1999.

[23] "Smartex Wearable Wellness System," (http://www.smartex.it/index.php/en/products/wearable-wellness-system), last access July 21, 2016.

[24] Y. He and Y. Li, "Physical activity recognition utilizing the built-in kinematic sensors of a smartphone," *International Journal of Distributed Sensor Networks*, vol. 9, no. 4, p. 481580, 2013.

[25] M. Zhang and A. A. Sawchuk, "A feature selection-based framework for human activity recognition using wearable multimodal sensors," in *Proceedings of the Sixth International Conference on Body Area Networks*. ICST (Institute for Computer Sciences, Social-Informatics and Telecommunications Engineering), 2011, pp. 92–98.

[26] G. Rescio, A. Leone, and P. Siciliano, "Supervised expert system for wearable MEMS accelerometer-based fall detector," *Journal of Sensors*, vol. 2013, 2013, pp. 11.

[27] Y. Gao, H. Qi, D.-y. Liu, and H. Liu, "Semi-supervised *k*-means clustering for multi-type relational data," in *International Conference on Machine Learning and Cybernetics*, vol. 1. San Diego, CA, IEEE, Dec. 2008, pp. 326–330.

[28] N. Noury and T. Hadidi, "Computer simulation of the activity of the elderly person living independently in a health smart home," *Computer Methods and Programs in Biomedicine*, vol. 108, no. 3, pp. 1216–1228, 2012.

[29] G. Virone, B. Lefebvre, N. Noury, and J. Demongeot, "Modeling and computer simulation of physiological rhythms and behaviors at home for data fusion programs in a telecare system," in *Proceedings of the Fifth International Workshop on Enterprise Networking and Computing in Healthcare Industry*. Santa Monica, CA, IEEE, Jun. 2003, pp. 111–117.

[30] L. Ljung, "Model validation and model error modelling," in *The Astrom Symposium on Control*, Lund, Sweden, 1999.

[31] R. A. Delgado, G. C. Goodwin, R. Carvajal, and J. C. Agüero, "A novel approach to model error modelling using the expectation-maximization algorithm," in *IEEE 51st Annual Conference on Decision and Control (CDC)*. Stuttgart, Germany, IEEE, Dec. 2012, pp. 7327–7332.

[32] Y. Zhao, B. Huang, H. Su, and J. Chu, "Prediction error method for identification of LPV models," *Journal of Process Control*, vol. 22, no. 1, pp. 180–193, 2012.

[33] S. Park and H. A. Kautz, "Privacy-preserving recognition of activities in daily living from multi-view silhouettes and RFID-based training." in *AAAI Fall Symposium: AI in Eldercare: New Solutions to Old Problems*, Menlo Park, CA, 2008, pp. 70–77.

[34] T. D. Nielsen and F. V. Jensen, *Bayesian Networks and Decision Graphs*. New York, Springer Science & Business Media, 2009.

[35] W. A. Barbakh, Y. Wu, and C. Fyfe, "Online clustering algorithms and reinforcement learning," in *Non-Standard Parameter Adaptation for Exploratory Data Analysis*. Berlin, Germany, Springer, 2009, pp. 85–108.

Chapter 7

Smart multi-sensor solutions for ADL detection

B. Andò, S. Baglio, C.O. Lombardo, and V. Marletta

Abstract

This chapter provides a review of the State of the Art in the Field of advanced solutions for the monitoring of critical events against elderly persons and people with neurological pathologies (e.g., Alzheimer's, Parkinson's). Many systems have been proposed in the literature which use cameras or other forms of sensing. Privacy, reliability and false alarms are the main challenges to be considered for the development of efficient systems to detect and classify the Activities of Daily Living (ADL) and Falls. The design of such systems, especially if wearable, requires a user centered design approach as well as the use of reliable sensors and advanced signal processing techniques, which have to fulfill constraints given by the power and computational budgets. As a case study, a solution based on a multi-sensor data fusion approach is presented. The system is able to recognize critical events like falls or prolonged inactivity and to detect the user posture. In particular, algorithms developed for the Activities of Daily Living classification combine data from an accelerometer and a gyroscope embedded in the user device. Tests performed on the developed prototype confirm the suitability of the device performances, which have been estimated in terms of sensitivity and specificity in performing Falls and ADL classification tasks. Apart from alerts management, the information provided by this system is useful to track the evolution of the user pathology, also during rehabilitation tasks.

7.1 Introduction

The need for Information and Communications Technology (ICT)-based solutions aimed to improve the life quality and autonomy of weak people, like elders or people with specific pathologies (e.g., Alzheimer's, Parkinson's), is really emerging. The scientific efforts of researchers working in this field can seriously affect the life of weak people in terms of well-being and active ageing. The involved environments range from hospitals to private homes.

In particular, this chapter focuses on the development of multi-sensor solutions to monitor the user activities during the everyday life: Activities of Daily Living (ADLs). ADLs are a wide set of actions characterizing the habits of people especially in their living places. User movements, stair negotiation, user posture, falls, sitting, standing up and lying down are just few examples of actions to be monitored. With particular regards to frail people with disabilities and elders, the monitoring of ADLs can produce a lot of information on their health status and critical events against themselves [1].

Falls are one of the main causes of injuries and trauma among elders, which can lead to extreme consequence especially in case of a delayed support from the caregiver. Approximately 37.3 million falls are severe enough to require medical attention each year, being age, gender and health of the individual can affect the type and severity of injury [2]. An estimated 424,000 fatal falls occur each year, which is the second leading cause of unintentional injury death.

Among risk factors causing falls effects of aging on gait, balance and strength, being confused and agitated, chronic diseases, medication side effects, incontinence, falls history (having fallen before), taking sedatives or sleeping tablets, behavioral symptoms and unsafe behaviors, environmental hazards, unsafe equipment, visual impairments are the most significant [3–7].

Although attempts of fall prevention can be performed by several activities, such as screening of living environments, clinical identification of risk factors, environmental assessment and adaptation and the use of assistive devices to address physical and sensory impairments, the reliable monitoring of ADLs and Falls would enable the possibility to achieve a real-time awareness on the user status and consequently to set actions aimed to fix the detected emergency. Moreover, minor falls can be detected which can anticipate future serious events. It must be considered that a reliable classification of falls could be strategic to assess daily rehabilitation and diagnostic tasks, especially for people with neurological diseases. The same assessment accomplished during clinical trials can suffer for serious user polarization and cannot be performed over a large observation time, also due to practical aspects.

In the next section a brief review of the state of art in the field of falls and ADL detection methodologies is presented, which highlights the need to fulfill mandatory features such as reliability, user acceptability and compliance with constraints due to the limited power budget and computational capability of wearable systems.

7.2 A review of the state of the art in fall detection systems

Different approaches have been proposed to detect ADLs and falls in the Ambient Assisted Living (AAL) context [8–33], such as customized devices [14–16] and smartphone-based platforms [17–24]. Other examples of fall detection and elderly monitoring systems are available in [25–28]. An extensive review of fall detection systems, including comparisons among different approaches, is available in [29]. Customized solutions, such as systems presented in [14–16], present sounding performances. Anyway, drawbacks of such systems are usually related to the users diffidence and discomfort (also due to the device positioning on the user body) and difficult to use. The trade-off between power budget and computational power could also represent a serious constraint, especially if wearable devices are under consideration.

Conversely to customized approaches, smartphone-based systems for ADLs detection can be considered convenient since no extra device is required and automatic dialing features are available. Many smartphone-based solutions for ADL monitoring are available in the literature, which exploits their intrinsic sensing and processing features [17–24]. A major problem with such approach seems to be the user acceptability, especially by elders, because of the need for training [17]. Moreover, another drawback is represented by the generation of false positives alerts due to smartphone manipulation by the user. Many efforts have been dedicated to develop smartphone-based ADL detectors which do not require user interaction, can be conveniently positioned on the user body and implements reliable ADL and fall detection algorithms. As an example, the possibility to use complex processing paradigms for downfall detection is investigated in [17]. An approach based on mobile phones and advanced signal processing for the monitoring of human physical activities, oriented to assist frail people is described in [18]. Investigation of human falls exploiting inertial sensors embedded in a smartphones is presented in [19]. The fall detection methodology illustrated in [20] is based on the exploitation of acceleration and orientation information gathered by smartphone sensors and processed by threshold algorithms. Different situations are taken into account: the smartphone is held by hand while typing SMS, the smartphone is next to the user's ear for listening and the smartphone is positioned in chest or pant pockets. In this work authors demonstrated that the methodology developed is capable of detecting and classifying three types of falls (forward, backward and aside) with good performances. Moreover, they demonstrated that no sitting or standing events were erroneously classified as falls while some other events, like walking and running-stop (indicated as ADL), were sometimes erroneously classified as fall.

An interesting approach for body movement analysis and classification, implemented through a waist-mounted smartphone is presented in [21]. A methodology allowing elders to live independently in their own homes, which is based on distributing sensors within the environment (Smart Home) and a cloud-based signal processing is investigated in [22]. In [23] authors present advanced paradigms to estimate trunk position during bipedal stance, in remote rehabilitation contexts. Features of a smartphone based approach for mobility monitoring, gaining awareness of changes-of-state caused by starting/stopping and postural change, are addressed in [29].

As evincible by the above state of the art and other related works in the literature [30–33] several methodologies use threshold algorithms applied to the user movement dynamics, while exploiting the information on the user posture before and after the estimated event. A different approach based on the use of cross-correlation between the user dynamics and fall/ADLs signatures is investigated in [10,11]. This approach is proposed by the research group working in the field of assistive technologies at the DIEEI of the University of Catania-Italy, which are currently involved in the development of innovative multi-sensor solutions for the monitoring of weak people (like elders or people with neurological pathologies) during their staying in social care or health facilities and nursing homes [34–36].

In [10] a smartphone-based platform for ADLs and fall detection is presented, which is able to acquire awareness of common ADLs, such as forward fall, backward fall, lateral fall, sitting down, stair negotiation and lying down, with the aim to implement recovery actions and to provide the user with a suitable degree of assistance. The proposed architecture uses advanced signal processing to detect ADLs, basically considering the moving average of the magnitude of the three acceleration components and event polarized cross-correlation analysis. The latter makes the system robust against anomalous dynamics. Two different threshold algorithms have been investigated for the sake of ADL classification. The first one is applied to the rough extracted features (maximum values of correlation between the unknown pattern and ADL signatures), while the other approach uses a threshold mechanism applied to a new data set obtained by a Principal Component Analysis (PCA).

In [11] an improvement of the classification methodology is presented. The classification methodology uses also the information on the user posture after the detected ADL, which allows for solving multiple classification of the same event. A large set of users has been used for paradigm tailoring (such as generating ADL signatures and fixing thresholds for the classification paradigms).

In [37] a data fusion strategy is used to improve the efficiency in Fall and ADLs classification as respect to [10,11]. The multisensor approach exploits data recorded from the accelerometer and gyroscope embedded in the device. A threshold mechanism is applied to features (maximum values of correlation between the unknown pattern and ADL and falls signatures) extracted from the moving average of the magnitude of the three acceleration components and angular velocities. As mentioned above, these information are then combined in order to reduce misclassifications, which can arise from two different cases: multiple classifications, i.e., the same unknown pattern is classified as belonging to several classes of events (low specificity) or wrong classifications, i.e., the pattern is recognized as belonging to the wrong class (low sensitivity). It must be noted that, conversely to fall detection systems using only the final user posture to recognize falls, which can fail due to extra movement of the user after the fall, the methodology proposed in [10,11,37] mainly analyzes the inertial signal evolution recorded during the fall event.

In the following section the system presented in [37] is deeply described, as a case study of a multisensor strategy to address the Fall/ADLs detection and classification task. The platform described could be exploited both for indoor and outdoor contexts, such as museums, hospitals, public sites but also for home use (e.g., the monitoring of patients recently discharged by the hospital).

7.3 Case study: a multisensor data fusion based fall detection system

The system developed for ADLs and falls detection uses a smartphone (user node) to be wear at the user hip, which is the most favorite position from the users point of view [37]. The device is equipped with the ultra-low-power/high performance/three-axes "nano" accelerometer, ST LIS3DH and the low-power three-axis gyroscope L3G4200D, both manufactured by ST Microelectronics. The accelerometer has dynamically user selectable full scales of ± 2 g/± 4 g/± 8 g/± 16 g, an output data rates ranging from 1 Hz to 5 kHz and a 16 bit output format provided by a I2C/SPI interface. The gyroscope has a full scale of ±250/±500/±2,000 dps, a user-selectable bandwidth (from 100 Hz to 800 Hz) and it is equipped with a I2C/SPI interface. Signals provided by the sensors are acquired with a sampling frequency of 50 Hz and stored on the SD card also for the sake of system debugging. Exploiting the communication facilities embedded in the smartphone, the information about the user posture and occurrence of critical events are easily conveyed to the caregiver.

The classes of falls and ADLs considered through this work are: forward fall (FF), backward fall (BF), lateral fall (LF), stair negotiation (step up by the right/left leg, 'SUR,L', step down 'SDR,L' by the right/left leg), lying down (LD) and sitting down (SI). As sketched in Figure 7.1, the methodology proposed is based on the consideration that above events are characterized by typical signatures in the time evolution of inertial quantities (acceleration and angular velocities) [11]. In order to extract features useful to classify an event as belonging to one of the above classes or not, maximum values of the cross-correlations between the inertial quantities measured for the unknown event and the set of signatures representative of the candidate ADLs are estimated. It must be considered that the use of a correlation-based analysis is strategic for the implementation of an event polarized classification paradigm, which is quite robust against exogenous dynamics. Such features are then processed through threshold algorithms to implement the event polarized classification approach. Successively, results provided by threshold algorithms applied to angular velocities and acceleration signals are conveyed to a data fusion paradigm to improve the robustness of the classification approach against misclassifications. In the following sections a brief review of the procedure adopted for the signature generation is presented, along

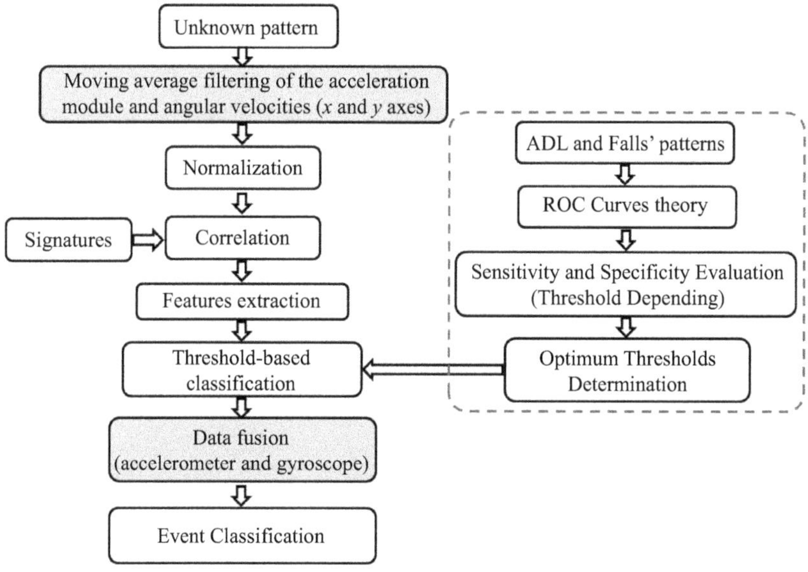

Figure 7.1 The classification approach (© [2016] IEEE)

with the implemented threshold algorithms and the data fusion approach adopted to filter out misclassifications.

7.3.1 Signal pre-processing and signature generation

The first step of the classification algorithm consists in performing a pre-processing of the acceleration magnitude and angular velocities by a moving average filter (working on time slots of 2 s shifted by 20 ms each other). Moreover, in order to compensate the gyroscope response for the misalignment of the smartphone (after the device has been worn by the user), with respect to the reference system shown in Figure 7.2, the initial values of the accelerometer components are acquired. Since the acceleration magnitude is considered, which is robust against the initial orientation of the device, only a standard bias and gain calibration of the accelerometer has been performed.

In order to make the classification procedure independent of the user characteristics (like height, weight, gender and ages), which can affect the acceleration magnitude and the angular velocities, a normalization procedure has been implemented both for the signatures and the inertial quantities measured for the unknown event. The normalization procedure fits signals in the range [−1, 1], thus preserving the signal's dynamics, while assuring the generalization of the classification strategy. This approach also increases the robustness of the system against light variations of the device position on the user body, as well as it reduces the need for a tuning phase, which would involve the user in performing simulated ADLs. For each class of ADLs a different set of normalization parameters was estimated.

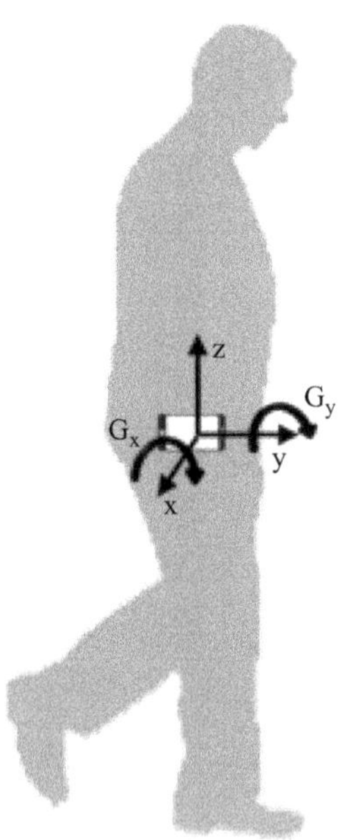

Figure 7.2 The reference system (© [2016] IEEE)

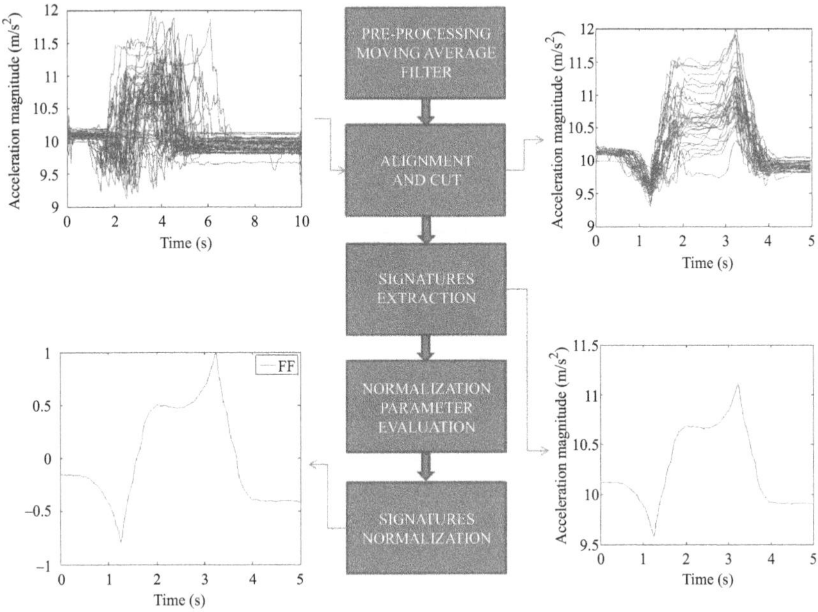

Figure 7.3 Methodology for the signatures generation. The example is related to the Forward Fall class (© [2015] IEEE)

The methodology adopted to generate signatures and schematized in Figure 7.3 is based on the creation of a dataset with several observations for each class of ADLs. For each observation, a time window of 10 s of the three acceleration components and of the two angular velocities has been recorded. For each set of events belonging to the same class, after the pre-processing step above discussed, the filtered signals (5 s time slot around the observed event) are aligned and averaged. The alignment algorithm uses both a threshold mechanism and the time delay between patterns, estimated by computing the cross-correlation between signals. It must be observed that the alignment procedure has been implemented only to extract signatures for each ADL, while this step is not required to classify the unknown event.

7.3.2 Features generation and threshold algorithms

As first, the unknown pattern (5 s time slots of acceleration and angular velocities) is pre-processed as described in Section 7.3.1. Successively, features (one per each of the nine candidate events for the three inertial quantities: nine for the acceleration magnitude, nine for the angular velocity along the x-axis and nine for the angular velocity along the y-axis) are extracted by computing maximum values of the cross-correlations between signals recorded in the time slot and the set of signatures representative of the candidate ADLs.

Three threshold classification algorithms compare the extracted features to threshold values: Accelerometer-based Threshold Algorithm (ATA), x-axis

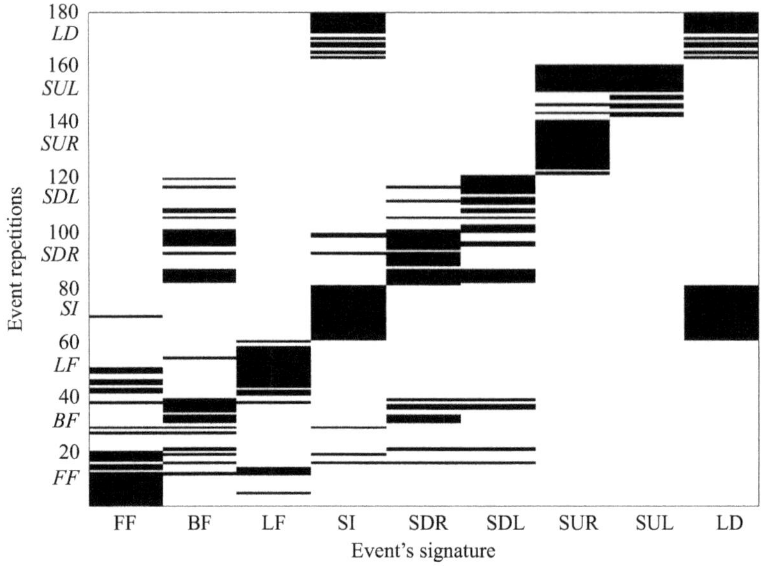

Figure 7.4 Results of event classification by the ATA classification algorithm for the test phase (© [2016] IEEE)

Gyroscope-based Threshold Algorithm (G_xTA) and y-axis Gyroscope-based Threshold Algorithm (G_yTA). Actually, an event is classified by each algorithm as potentially belonging to a specific class if its correlation with the corresponding signature exceeds the pre-defined threshold. To define the optimal threshold values, the Receiver Operating Characteristic (ROC) theory was used.[1]

Outputs from threshold algorithms ATA, G_xTA and G_yTA are the matrixes $R^{Acc}_{(0,1)i,j}$, $R^{Gyr,x}_{(0,1)i,j}$ and $R^{Gyr,y}_{(0,1)i,j}$ (where i states for a generic time slot and $j = 1:9$ states for the candidate events). Each element can be 1 or 0, depending if the corresponding feature exceeds the related threshold or not.

As an example the map $R^{Acc}_{(0,1)i,j}$, shown in Figure 7.4, was obtained by applying the ATA algorithm to a set of 180 unknown patterns, obtained by repeating 20 experiments

[1]The ROC approach confers the possibility to improve the system sensitivity at the extent of the system selectivity and vice versa, in the respect of constraints driven by the specific application. In real problems the best case rarely exists, i.e., two classes are perfectly separated with a well-defined cut-off value. Indeed, a situation with an overlap between two classes (positive and negative classes) is typically observed. The ROC curves theory provides a theoretical support to the classification problem where a classifier is required to map each instance (i.e., event to classify) to one of the two classes [38,39]. For every possible threshold value adopted to discriminate between two populations of events, the True Positive Rate (*TPR*) or Sensitivity and the True Negative Rate (*TNR*) or Specificity can be evaluated. An ROC curve is a 2D plot of the *TPR* (Sensitivity) vs. the False Positive Rate defined as $FPR = 1$-Specificity for a binary classifier system, as its discrimination threshold varies [40,41].

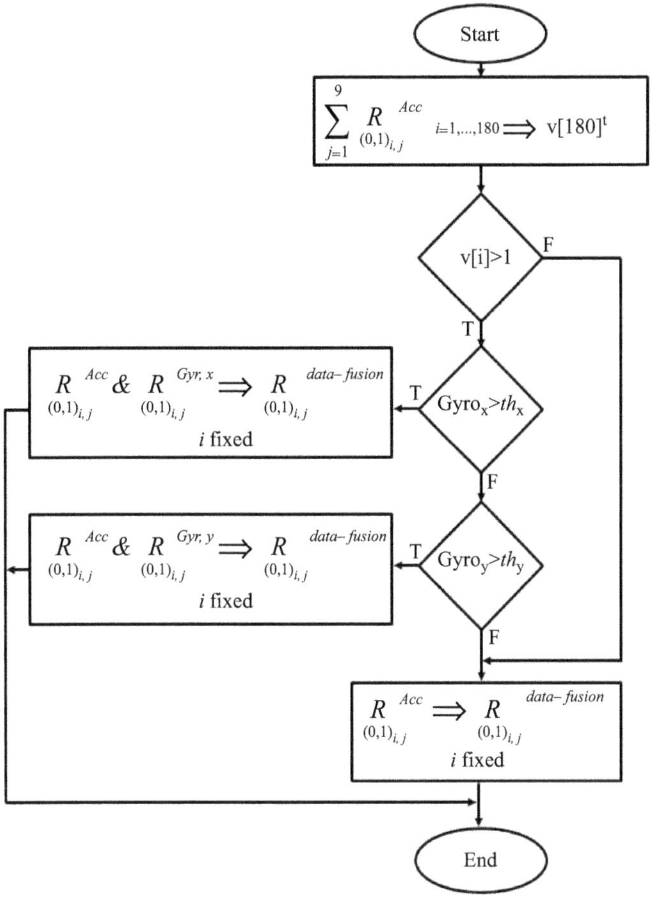

Figure 7.5 The multi-sensor Data Fusion paradigm for ADL and Fall detection. For the case developed, 20 repetitions (time slots) for each of the nine events have been considered (© [2016] IEEE)

for each of the nine classes of events. The horizontal axis shows the event classes, while repeated events for each class are reported in the vertical axis. Black cells correspond to recognized (correctly or not) events.

As can be observed by the map shown in Figure 7.4, three cases are possible: the event is correctly classified as belonging only to its nominal class; the event is classified as belonging to several classes including its nominal class (multiple classification); the event is classified as belonging to wrong classes, not including its nominal class (wrong classifications). Above occurrences produce misclassifications leading to false positive and false negative estimations.

In order to improve the reliability of the classification task the multi-sensor data fusion paradigm, shown in Figure 7.5, has been used. In case a multiple classification is obtained by the ATA Algorithm, the corresponding G_x component of the Gyroscope is analyzed. If the maximum value of the normalized amplitude is higher than a threshold (heuristically fixed to 0.3 on the basis of a wide set of data obtained during the experimental sessions with real users), such component is considered meaningful and the results of the G_xTA algorithm are combined by a logic AND operator with the results obtained by the ATA. Otherwise, the above operation is repeated to the result of the G_yTA algorithm, by using the same heuristic value of the threshold.

The approach adopted to implement the constrained logic combination of results provided by the ATA, G_xTA and G_yTA algorithms is briefly summarized in the following notes. Starting from the results provided by the ATA, all the columns of $R^{Acc}_{(0,1)i,j}$ are added together thus obtaining a new column vector, C^{Acc}_i (its dimension is 180 with reference to the matrix in Figure 7.5). Each element of C^{Acc}_i (corresponding to an unknown event to be classified) is then processed. If the value of a generic element, C^{Acc}_q of C^{Acc}_i is not greater than 1 (the event was classified as belonging to only one class of events or none), the related row, q, of $R^{Acc}_{(0,1)i,j}$ is copied without modifications in the new matrix $R^{data\text{-}fusion}_{(0,1)i,j}$. The latter represents the final matrix used for the classification task. If the value of C^{Acc}_q is greater than 1 (the event was classified as belonging to several classes), the x component of the gyroscope output is evaluated. In case the maximum of the normalized signal in the 5 s time slot exceeds a threshold the related row, q, of $R^{Acc}_{(0,1)i,j}$ is combined by a logic AND operator with the corresponding row of $R^{Gyr,x}_{(0,1)i,j}$. The resulting row is then inserted in the cross-correlation matrix $R^{data\text{-}fusion}_{(0,1)i,j}$. In case the G_x component results meaningless in the considered time window, the same procedure is applied to the G_y component of the gyroscope output and the $R^{Gyr,x}_{(0,1)i,j}$ cross-correlation matrix. In case the two conditions on the two axes of the gyroscope are not satisfied, the q row of $R^{Acc}_{(0,1)i,j}$ is copied to $R^{data\text{-}fusion}_{(0,1)i,j}$.

7.3.3 The experimental validation of the classification methodology by end users

As a necessary premise it must be observed that, although users addressed by the solution developed are elders and people with neurological diseases, for safety reasons the system has been tested by using standard manikin and successively by users in good shape. During the experiments all the precautions have been taken to avoid injuries. To support the validity of the test performed, it must be considered that the cross-correlation classification algorithms is robust against light modifications of unknown patterns and the classification procedure can be successfully applied to a new set of signatures (generated by real users). The characteristics of the users involved in the tests are summarized in Table 7.1.

Each user was requested to repeat five actions for all the classes of events considered. Repetitions from six users (30 patterns per each event) were used, during the learning phase, to extract the signatures and the normalization parameters for each kind of event. The repetitions from the other four users (20 patterns per each event)

Table 7.1 Characteristics of the users involved in the tests (© [2015] IEEE)

Gender	**USER1 Male**	**USER2 Male**	**USER3 Female**	**USER4 Male**	**USER5 Male**	**USER6 Female**	**USER7 Male**	**USER8 Male**	**USER9 Female**	**USER10 Male**
Age (year)	36	25	40	36	31	44	40	36	39	42
Height (m)	1.75	1.85	1.62	1.78	1.66	1.54	1.81	1.65	1.58	1.92
Weight (kg)	90	82	54	85	72	52	81	63	60	105

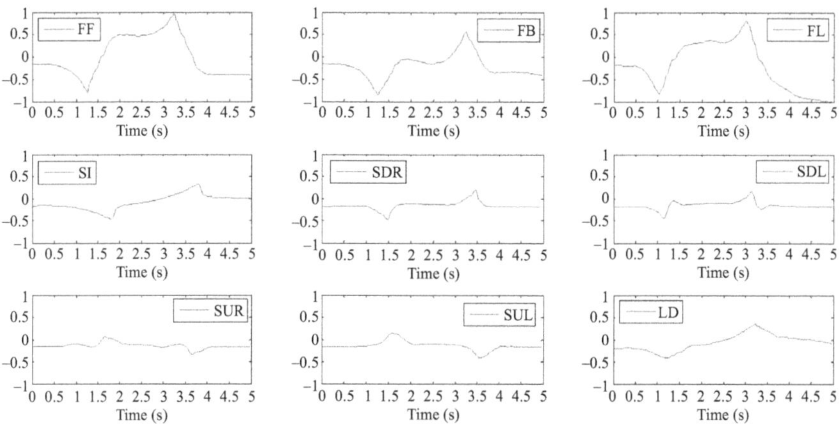

Figure 7.6 Normalized signatures for each class of events generated by the learning data set of the acceleration signal (© [2015] IEEE)

were used during the test phase to extract features. As an example, the estimated signatures for the acceleration signals are shown in Figure 7.6, while Table 7.2 shows the maximum cross-correlation between 10 FF events and all the set of signatures for the acceleration signal.

Although high correlation with the FF signature emerges, noticeable correlation values can be also obtained by correlating the unknown pattern to other signatures. Processing such results by the ATA algorithm leads to results shown in Figure 7.4. Threshold values for the ATA algorithm are given in Table 7.3.

As can be observed, a number of multiple classifications were obtained where the same event is classified as belonging to different classes. Moreover, there are events which are wrongly classified as belonging to another class. Such behavior leads to the generation of misclassifications which produce False Positives and False Negatives.

Performances of the classification paradigms have been estimated by means of the following indexes:

$$Sensitivity = \frac{TP}{TP + FN} \tag{7.1}$$

Table 7.2 Correlations between each signature and ten patterns, used during the learning phase, corresponding to the forward fall event (© [2016] IEEE)

FF	BF	LF	SI	SDR	SDL	SUR	SUL	LD
0.9339	0.7754	0.7530	0.6286	0.5447	0.5540	0.2841	0.3980	0.6839
0.8490	0.3984	0.5953	0.3782	0.1133	0.1370	0.0926	0.0852	0.4835
0.9492	0.7173	0.7724	0.5983	0.4551	0.5053	0.2259	0.2646	0.6114
0.9188	0.5276	0.6782	0.4788	0.2201	0.2585	0.1597	0.1528	0.5490
0.9058	0.6853	0.8410	0.5217	0.4627	0.5545	0.2669	0.4371	0.5870
0.9167	0.6856	0.7899	0.5532	0.4467	0.5191	0.2121	0.3037	0.5586
0.8761	0.4371	0.6257	0.4087	0.1381	0.1636	0.1074	0.0990	0.5019
0.8791	0.4510	0.6720	0.3860	0.1986	0.2153	0.1437	0.1358	0.5074
0.8563	0.3963	0.5968	0.3708	0.1171	0.1462	0.0921	0.0858	0.4780
0.8930	0.5392	0.7008	0.4498	0.2666	0.3281	0.1681	0.1836	0.5329

Table 7.3 Thresholds estimated by the ROC curve during the learning phase for the ATA classification paradigm (© [2016] IEEE)

FF	BF	LF	SI	SDR	SDL	SUR	SUL	LD
0.7705	0.7795	0.7941	0.7793	0.8803	0.8954	0.9094	0.9463	0.8374

Table 7.4 Sensitivity and specificity features for the ATA and data fusion classification paradigm (© [2016] IEEE)

	ATA		Data fusion	
	Sensitivity	**Specificity**	**Sensitivity**	**Specificity**
FF	0.90	0.94	0.90	1.00
BF	0.55	0.86	0.55	0.99
LF	0.90	0.97	0.90	0.99
SI	1.00	0.88	0.95	0.98
SDR	0.90	0.93	0.90	0.98
SDL	0.75	0.92	0.75	0.95
SUR	0.95	0.93	0.95	0.93
SUL	0.80	1.00	0.80	1.00
LD	0.70	0.88	0.60	1.00

$$Specificity = \frac{TN}{TN + FP} \tag{7.2}$$

where TP, TN, FP and FN, stand for True Positives, True Negatives, False Positives and False Negatives, respectively. Results obtained in terms of specificity and sensitivity in case of the ATA algorithm are given in Table 7.4. As an example, the BF classification suffers for a low specificity.

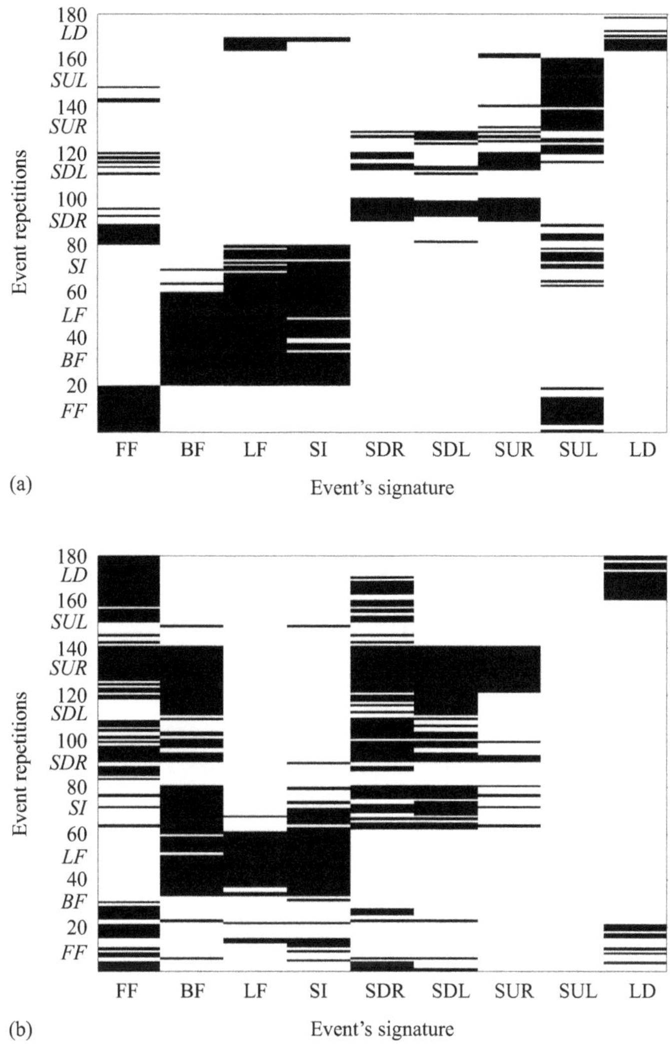

Figure 7.7 Results of event classification by the (a) G_xTA and (b) G_yTA algorithms for the test phase (© [2016] IEEE)

In order to reduce misclassifications, the G_xTA and G_yTA algorithms have been used. Results for the considered data set are shown in Figure 7.7, with the threshold given in Table 7.5. Results obtained in terms of specificity and sensitivity, after the application of the proposed data fusion algorithm are given in Table 7.4. The graphical representation of $R^{data\text{-}fusion}_{(0,1)_{i,j}}$, shown in Figure 7.8, evidences the performances of the data fusion classification algorithm in terms of misclassifications reduction, thus allowing for properly recognizing different classes of falls and ADL activities.

Table 7.5 Thresholds estimated by the ROC curves during the learning phase for the GXTA, GYTA classification paradigm (© [2016] IEEE)

	FF	BF	LF	SI	SDR	SDL	SUR	SUL	LD
Gyr,x	0.6932	0.9707	0.9102	0.9618	0.8857	0.8765	0.8248	0.5290	0.9576
Gyr.y	0.6307	0.7375	0.9751	0.7805	0.7379	0.7913	0.9308	0.8348	0.9404

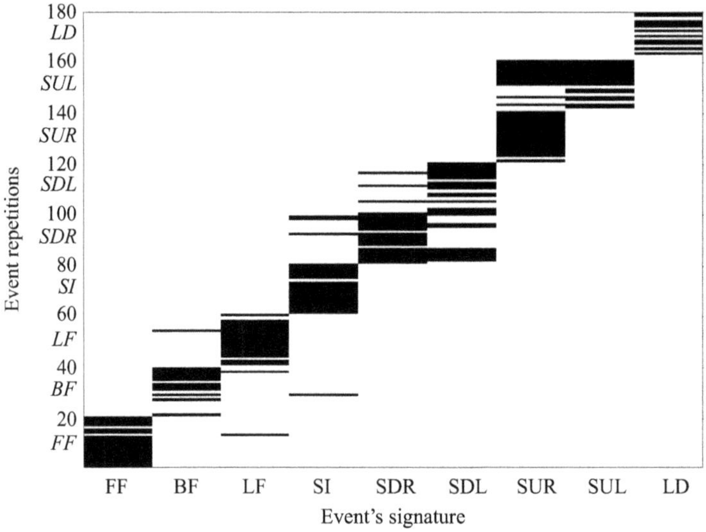

Figure 7.8 Results of event classification by the data fusion algorithm (© [2016] IEEE)

7.4 Conclusions

This chapter deals with a review of ADL and Fall detection systems, which are particularly relevant to cope with needs of elderly and users with neurological disorders.

The case study presented focuses on a novel methodology for ADLs classification, with particular regards to Fall events. In particular, the performances of a smartphone based multi-sensor data fusion approach, combining data from the onboard accelerometer and gyroscope, has been presented. The proposed approach allows for separating falls from other ADLs and to classify among different kind of falls, which is relevant in case of remote monitoring of elderly and impaired people and to perform diagnostic or rehabilitation tasks. From a methodological point of view, the solution adopted for Fall and ADL classification is mainly based on the analysis of the inertial signal evolution during the fall event and its correlation with known signatures, which make the system robust against artifacts. Moreover, the normalization procedure adopted makes the system insensitive against the strength of the acceleration signal, which is strictly correlated to the user characteristics (e.g., the height or the weight). The above strategies allow for a high specificity and sensibility in terms of ADLs classification, with a dramatic reduction of misclassification and consequently false alarms. Finally the system developed implements a complete automatic event detection and caregiver notification strategy, which is mandatory to avoid delay in performing the emergency procedure and implementing the recovery actions.

References

[1] I.D. Cameron, L.D. Gillespie, M.C. Robertson, *et al.*, Interventions for preventing falls in older people in care facilities and hospitals (Review), *Cochrane Database of Systematic Reviews*, London, UK, Wiley & Sons, Issue 12, 2012.

[2] World Health Organization, Falls, Fact sheet No. 344 [online], 2012. Available from: http://www.who.int/mediacentre/factsheets/fs344/en/ [Accessed August 2016].

[3] National Institute for Health and Clinical Excellence, 2013. Falls in older people: assessing risk and prevention [online]. Available from: http://www.nice.org.uk/guidance/cg161 [Accessed August 2016].

[4] Agency for Healthcare Research and Quality, The Falls Management Program: A Quality Improvement Initiative for Nursing Facilities, 2014. Available from: http://www.ahrq.gov/professionals/systems/long-term-care/resources/injuries/fallspx/index.html [Accessed August 2016].

[5] Agency for Healthcare Research and Quality, Module 3: Falls Prevention and Management, 2014. Available from: http://www.ahrq.gov/professionals/systems/long-term-care/resources/facilities/ptsafety/ltcmodule3.html [Accessed August 2016].

[6] R. Schwendimann, "Patient falls: a key issue in patient safety in hospitals", *PhD dissertation*, University of Basel, Faculty of Science, 2006. Available from: http://edoc.unibas.ch/495/1/DissB_7645.pdf [Accessed August 2016].

[7] P. Halfon, Y. Eggli, G. Van_Melle, A. Vagnair, "Risk of falls for hospitalized patients: a predictive model based on routinely available data", *Journal of Clinical Epidemiology*, 2001, 54(12):1258–66.

[8] N.K. Suryadevara, S.C. Mukhopadhyay, "Wireless sensor network based home monitoring system for wellness determination of elderly", *IEEE Sensors Journal*, 2012, 12(6):1965–72.

[9] B. Andò, S. Baglio, C.O. Lombardo, V. Marletta, "A multi-user assistive system for the user safety monitoring in care facilities", *Proceedings of the IEEE International Workshop on Measurement and Networking*, M&N 2015, Coimbra, Portugal, October 2015, pp. 1–5.

[10] B. Andò, S. Baglio, C.O. Lombardo, V. Marletta, E.A. Pergolizzi, A. Pistorio, "An event polarized paradigm for ADL detection in AAL context", *Proceedings of the IEEE International Instrumentation and Measurement Technology Conference (I2MTC)*, Montevideo, Uruguay, May 2014, pp. 1079–82.

[11] B. Andò, S. Baglio, C.O. Lombardo, V. Marletta, "An event polarized paradigm for ADL detection in AAL context", *IEEE Transactions on Instrumentation and Measurement*, 2015, 64(7):1814–25.
[12] E. Lou, N.G. Durdle, V.J. Raso, D.L. Hill, "A low-power posture measurement system for the treatment of scoliosis", *IEEE Transactions on Instrumentation and Measurement*, 2000, 49(1):108–13.
[13] Wai-Yin Wong, Man-Sang Wong, "Measurement of postural change in trunk movements using three sensor modules", *IEEE Transactions on Instrumentation and Measurement*, 2009, 58(8):2737–42.
[14] G. Rescio, A. Leone, P. Siciliano, "Supervised expert system for wearable MEMS accelerometer-based fall detector", *Journal of Sensors*, 2013, Article ID 254629, 11 pages.
[15] G. Panahandeh, N. Mohammadiha, A. Leijon, P. Handel, "Chest-mounted inertial measurement unit for pedestrian motion classification using continuous hidden Markov model", *Proceedings of the IEEE International Instrumentation and Measurement Technology Conference (I2MTC)*, Graz, Austria, May 2012, pp. 991–5.
[16] J.M. Kang, T. Yoo, H.C. Kim, "A wrist-worn integrated health monitoring instrument with a tele-reporting device for telemedicine and telecare", *IEEE Transactions on Instrumentation and Measurement*, 2006, 55(5):1655–61.
[17] J. Dunkel, R. Bruns, S. Stipkovic, "Event-based smartphone sensor processing for ambient assisted living", *Proceedings of the 11th IEEE International Symposium on Autonomous Decentralized Systems (ISADS)*, Mexico City, Mexico, March 2013, pp. 1–6.
[18] H. Ketabdar, M. Lyra, "System and methodology for using mobile phones in live remote monitoring of physical activities", *Proceedings of the IEEE International Symposium on Technology and Society (ISTAS)*, Wollongong, NSW, June 2010, pp. 350–6.
[19] C. Tacconi, S. Mellone, L. Chiari, "Smartphone-based applications for investigating falls and mobility", *Proceedings of the Fifth International Conference on Pervasive Computing Technologies for Healthcare (PervasiveHealth) and Workshops*, Dublin, Ireland, May 2011, pp. 258–61.
[20] V.Q. Viet, G. Lee, D. Choi, "Fall detection based on movement and smart phone technology", *Proceedings of the IEEE International Conference on Computing and Communication Technologies, Research, Innovation, and Vision for the Future (RIVF)*, Ho Chi Minh City, Vietnam, February 27–March 1 2012, pp. 1–4.
[21] Y. He, Y. Li, S. Bao, "Fall detection by built-in tri-accelerometer of smartphone", *Proceedings of the IEEE-EMBS International Conference on Biomedical and Health Informatics (BHI)*, Hong Kong, January 2012, pp. 184–7.
[22] M. Fahim, I. Fatima, S. Lee, Y. Lee, "Daily life activity tracking application for smart homes using android smartphone", *Proceedings of the 14th International Conference on Advanced Communication Technology (ICACT)*, PyeongChang, South Korea, February 2012, pp. 241–5.

[23] C. Franco, A. Fleury, P.Y. Gumery, B. Diot, J. Demongeot, N. Vuillerme, "iBalance-ABF: a smartphone-based audio-biofeedback balance system", *IEEE Transactions on Biomedical Engineering*, 2013, 60(1):211–5.

[24] G. Hache, E.D. Lemaire, N. Baddour, "Mobility change-of-state detection using a smartphone-based approach", *Proceedings of the IEEE International Workshop on Medical Measurements and Applications (MeMeA)*, Ottawa, ON, April 30–May 1, 2010, pp. 43–6.

[25] M. Kangas, A. Konttila, P. Lindgren, I. Winblad, T. Jämsä, "Comparison of low-complexity fall detection algorithms for body attached accelerometers", *Gait Posture*, 2008, 28(2):285–91.

[26] M. Kangas, A. Konttila, I. Winblad, T. Jämsä, "Determination of simple thresholds for accelerometry-based parameters for fall detection", *Proceedings of the 29th Annual International Conference of the IEEE Engineering in Medicine and Biology Society (EMBS)*, Lyon, France, August 2007, pp. 1367–70.

[27] M. Anwar Hossain, D. Tanvir Ahmed, "Virtual caregiver: an ambient-aware elderly monitoring system", *IEEE Transactions on Information Technology in Biomedicine*, 2012, 16(6):1024–31.

[28] J.C. Castillo, D. Carneiro, J. Serrano-Cuerda, P. Novais, A. Fernndez-Caballero, J. Neves, "A multi-modal approach for activity classification and fall detection", *International Journal of Systems Science*, 2014, 45(4):810–24.

[29] R. Igual, C. Medrano, I. Plaza, "Challenges, issues and trends in fall detection systems", *BioMedical Engineering OnLine*, 2013, 12(66), pp. 1–24. Available from: http://www.biomedical-engineering-online.com/content/12/1/66 [Accessed 16 August 2016].

[30] A.K. Bourke, G.M. Lyons, "A threshold-based fall detection algorithm using a bi-axial gyroscope sensor", *Medical Engineering and Physics*, 2008, 30(1): 84–90.

[31] A. K. Bourke, J. V. O'Brien, G. M. Lyons, "Evaluation of a threshold-based tri-axial accelerometer fall detection algorithm", *Gait Posture*, 2007, 26(2): 194–9.

[32] Q. Li, J.A. Stankovic, M.A. Hanson, A.T. Barth, J. Lach, G. Zhou, "Accurate, fast fall detection using gyroscopes and accelerometer-derived posture information", *Proceedings of the Sixth IEEE International Workshop on Wearable and Implantable Body Sensor Networks (BSN)*, Berkeley, CA, June 2009, pp. 138–143.

[33] H. Kerdegari, K. Samsudin, A.R. Ramli, S. Mokaram, "Evaluation of fall detection classification approaches", *Proceedings of the Fourth IEEE International Conference on Intelligent and Advanced Systems (ICIAS)*, Kuala Lumpur, Malaysia, June 2012, pp. 131–6.

[34] B. Andò, A. Ascia, "Navigation aids for the visually impaired: from artificial codification to natural sensing", *IEEE Magazine on Instrumentation and Measurements*, 2007, 10(3):44–51.

[35] B. Andò, N. Savalli, "CANBUS networked sensors use in orientation tools for the visually impaired wired versus wireless technology", *IEEE Magazine on Instrumentation and Measurements*, 2008, 11(1):49–52.

[36] B. Andò, S. Baglio, S. La Malfa, V. Marletta, "A sensing architecture for mutual user-environment awareness case of study: a mobility aid for the visually impaired", *IEEE Sensor Journal*, 2011, 11(3):634–40.
[37] B. Andò, S. Baglio, C.O. Lombardo, V. Marletta, "A multisensor data-fusion approach for ADL and Fall classification", *IEEE Transactions on Instrumentation and Measurement*, 2016, 65(9):1960–7.
[38] T. Fawcett, ROC graphs: notes and practical considerations for data mining researchers, *HP Technical Report HPL-2003-4*, HP Laboratories, 2003.
[39] A. Slaby, "ROC Analysis with Matlab", *Proceedings of the 29th International Conference on Information Technology Interfaces (ITI)*, Cavtat, Croatia, June 2007, pp. 191–6.
[40] D. Hand, R.J. Till, "A simple generalisation of the area under the ROC curve for multiple class classification", *Machine Learning*, 2001, 45(2):171–86.
[41] Z.-C. Qin, 'ROC analysis for predictions made by probabilistic classifiers", *Proceedings of the Fourth International Conference on Machine Learning and Cybernetics*, Guangzhou, China, vol. 5, August 2005, pp. 3119–24.

Chapter 8

Comprehensive human monitoring based on heterogeneous sensor network

Valentina Bianchi, Ferdinando Grossi, Claudio Guerra, Niccolò Mora, Agostino Losardo, Guido Matrella, Ilaria De Munari, and Paolo Ciampolini

Abstract

Healthcare paradigms, due to demographic changes, are definitely aiming at effective prevention and early diagnosis strategies. This inherently calls for continuous monitoring of (ageing) people in their own living environment and while attending at daily living activities. Such monitoring may rely on a wide range of sensing technologies, each featuring different trade-offs among main parameters such as accuracy, expressivity, cost, reliability and intrusively. This includes clinical sensors (suitable for self-managed, precise measurement of physiological parameters), wearable devices (continuously monitoring health or activity features) and environmental sensors distributed in the living environment (suitable for indirect assessment of relevant behaviours, besides serving basic safety purposes). In this chapter, the meaning of human monitoring from a home-care point of view will be defined, and the basic sensor categories will be reviewed. Then, the design and the main features of the CARDEA home monitoring system will be discussed. Finally, some application examples, coming from European project living-lab experiences, will be illustrated, and some results obtained by data fusion and analysis techniques, suitable for inferring health and wellness information by effectively correlating raw data coming from the sensor field, will be presented.

8.1 Introduction

Unprecedented demographic changes are affecting the main industrialized countries, and Europe in particular, depending on: population ageing, low birth rates, changes in family structures and migration [1]. Reports and projections from European Union are available, covering the period up to 2080 [2], to support the European governments in facing such scenario by developing suitable strategies and policies. Among many relevant concerns, population ageing mostly impact on healthcare and long-term care issues [3].

In this perspective, healthcare provision paradigms need to shift from traditional services models, mainly based on hospitalization in dedicated facilities, towards homecare services, which offer a number of significant advantages. By allowing elderly people to stay longer in their own homes, their habits and lifestyle can be preserved and their supporting network (relative, friends, caregivers) can be more effectively involved. Besides preserving individual quality-of-life indicators, a more efficient use of economic resources can be pursued as well, possibly reducing the burden on care institutions and services.

ICTs (Information and Communication Technologies) can foster and facilitate the improvement of homecare services in many different ways. For instance, by enabling effective prevention and early diagnosis strategies, by increasing social relation, by improving home safety, by tracking home activity and detecting anomalies [4]. Among ICT contribution to such new healthcare scenarios, human monitoring techniques are discussed in this chapter.

In the following subsections, the main enabling technologies are first reviewed, with particular regards to the basic categories of sensors and devices. Then, data fusion and analysis techniques (suitable for inferring health and wellness information from raw data coming from environmental monitoring) are introduced. As an example, the architecture of the CARDEA [5] system is presented. To provide a practical example, outcomes of the Helicopter AAL-JP Project [6] are discussed, based on a heterogeneous sensors network and tested in real-world environments, through transnational pilot experiences.

Eventually, some conclusions are drawn in the final section.

8.2 Human monitoring

In the context of this chapter, by "continuous human monitoring" we refer to the possibility, enabled by ICTs, of measuring a set of heterogeneous (i.e. not necessarily clinical) parameters in order to get information about the user's health, wellness and safety within his living environment (typically, his own home).

A number of physiological parameters can be easily obtained by means of clinical devices, suitable for home use and enabling self-assessment of parameters such as body weight, blood pressure, glycaemia and blood oxygen concentration. Telemedicine approaches rely on systematic acquisition and remote monitoring of such parameters. Therefore, they inherently depend on end-user scrupulousness in complying with the given schedule: this, however, may be perceived as a boring and intrusive task, and can possibly be jeopardized by cognitive or memory issues. Moreover, the clinical view provided by telemedicine practices is constrained by the time-discrete intervals of the assessment and by the limited availability of self-manageable devices (which inherently yields a low dimensionality of the acquired picture). Increasing both dimensionality and continuity can be achieved by complementing telemedicine data with further sensor information: in fact, many health issues may be inferred from "behavioural symptoms" (such as changes in feeding or sleeping patterns, physical activity, toilet frequency) which can be assessed by means of indirect indicators. They are, of course, not reliable enough for actual clinical diagnosis, but may provide early detection of anomalies, addressing the user, or the caregivers, towards more accurate assessment.

In this view, looking for behavioural features within the home environment may provide relevant information. Quantitative assessment may be carried out, as well as a qualitative one, involving recognition of the actual kind of activity carried out. Detection and recognition of Activities of Daily Living (ADL: eating, walking, cooking, etc.) is a challenging task indeed: a notable example of possible application consists of fall detection: many systems, sensors and algorithms have been developed, in recent year, to cope with this emergency condition.

The use of an ICT-based continuous human monitoring can yield benefits for different stakeholders: end-users, informal and formal caregivers, local care service providers, public health systems.

Elderly users, for example, can enjoy a better safety feeling, coming from the perception of being continually monitored. Environmental monitoring can be exploited also for safety and security purposes. Furthermore, the use of accessible and familiar technologies, such as smartphones, can be exploited to provide advices and tips, coaching towards the adoption of healthier lifestyles (regular intake of medication, personalized diet, exercises for physical or cognitive activities).

Caregivers may take advantage of the ICT-based continuous monitoring by obtaining "objective" information and data related to users' behaviour, suitable for being correlated to their subjective perceptions, thus providing a more comprehensive pictures, and to evaluate effects of care actions on user's activity and health. Data analytics (providing, for instance, trend analysis) also allows to detect phenomena which could remain unnoticed otherwise (for instance, decrease in motion activity slowly varying in time). The same information can also be useful to care providers to improve the service performance: for example, by changing dynamically the priorities of service delivery according to the actual needs of users, as assessed through monitoring.

Similarly, public health systems can take advantage of more detailed and continuous knowledge about the user health in order to optimize the care provision policies. Monitoring support prevention and early diagnosis, this possibly resulting in more effective cure and in decreasing hospitalization costs.

8.3 Technology overview

The fields of human monitoring, smart health and ambient/active assisted living actually share similar technology foundations, and are often mixed and integrated in a common context, with the same information possibly being exploited with different goals.

A detailed cataloguing of such background technologies goes beyond the scope of this work: many excellent reviews can be found in the technical literature [7–11]. In the following, a short summary of relevant application features is given.

ADLs recognition. "Activities of Daily Living" is an expression used to indicate people's daily self-care tasks. The purpose of the recognition is to detect activities such as feeding, bathing, dressing, sleeping, cooking, relaxing, working and any other activities a person usually does during his day. Automatic recognition of ADLs can enable behavioural analyses, suitable for coaching purposes and for anomaly and trend detection. To achieve a reliable ADL detection different approach are used, exploiting environmental sensors, or wearable mobile sensors (smartphones or smart bracelets). Cameras can be used as well. All sensors produce raw data which need to be suitably interpreted to infer ADL information. This calls for reliable processing and classification, often based on artificial intelligence techniques [12–14].

Localization and identification. The knowledge of how user uses his living environments helps to define the context and the habits of his life. Hence, several techniques aiming at localizing a person inside his home environment have been devised [15]. Whenever more than one single person inhabits the home, a further problem arises, consisting of the need of recognizing the user actually interacting with a given sensor. Identification techniques are needed to this purpose [16].

Anomaly and trend detection. Based on ADLs recognition and localization, further processing can be performed at a higher abstraction level, implementing Behavioural Analysis capability. Analysing the way (e.g. duration, frequency and other features of specific tasks) in which the user performs his ADLs, anomalies (i.e. meaningful deviations from the usual behaviour) and trends (drifts in usual behavioural patterns) can be detected [17].

Health monitoring. In order to ensure an early detection of illness symptoms, a frequent monitoring of user's physiological parameter is desirable. Clinical sensors suitable for telemedicine applications are available, featuring user-friendliness and communication capabilities (mostly based on Bluetooth technology) which allows for integrating into more general monitoring or AAL systems [18].

Planning and coaching. The increasingly widespread use of smartphone and tablet, even among elderly people, enable to implement APPs interfacing to the monitoring systems and providing users with useful feedback. For instance, supporting the user in managing their daily schedule (taking medications, for instance) or providing them with context- and behaviour-sensitive advices, coaching towards a healthier lifestyle [19–21].

Environmental and personal safety. Technologies developed in order to monitor personal and environmental safety are quite diffused and often associated to homecare and assistive applications. Hazards such as gas leaks, flooding, fires can be detected using available sensors [22,23]. Smart solutions have been devised to recognize more specific risks, regarding in particular elderly persons: fall detection and prevention can be implemented [24], as well as wandering behaviour [25].

To implement the above features, technologies are needed. Main technologies used in the assistive and AAL frameworks include:

Smart Home. With this expression we refer to a home in which technologies like IoT (Internet of Things) and AI (Ambient Intelligence) are exploited to implement home monitor and control services [26,27]. The variety of devices which can be considered is virtually unlimited. A non-exhaustive list of most popular devices includes:

- PIR (passive infra-red) sensors. Wall-mounted devices that detect the motion of a person in the room. Typically used in security systems or for automation purposes (e.g., to turn on the lights automatically). Distributed throughout the home, they can be used to monitor and track the movement of users inside the home.
- Switch and remote controls. Mobile switches allow a more comfortable control of lights and home automation (e.g. blinds, shutters, curtains, or simple household appliances). They also can be used to provide the monitoring system with information on user habits.
- Occupancy sensors. Implemented by means of a different technology (pressure pads, proximity sensors, microphones, cameras, etc.), they provide information about the user being located at a specific location, relevant to behaviour monitoring (e.g., the bed, toilet).
- Open/close sensor. Typically, are magnetic contacts used to detect if a door (or a window, a drawer, a furniture door, etc.) is open or closed. If installed on the perimeters doors (or windows) of the users' home, it may serve security purposes. If installed on a particular spot (e.g. the medicine cabinet, or the fridge), it can be used to monitor health-related behaviours as well.
- Power outlet monitoring sensor. Smart plugs enable the measurement of instant electrical power consumption. They allow to infer when a given appliance (e.g. the TV set) is being used and can be included in behavioural tracking applications.

Wearable sensors. Devices worn by the user, suitable for evaluating physical activity, as well as to assess in a continuous fashion basic physiological data (e.g. heartbeat rate, body temperature) developed to measure specific parameter related to the movement of persons within the home environment. They have a crucial role to achieve also contribute to localization functions, user identification, and fall detection purposes [28,29].

Clinical sensors. Aimed at measuring quantities such as bodyweight, blood pressure, glucose, oxygen concentration.

Robotics. Service robots can be exploited in many different ways; in the current vision, besides ADL support, robots can be used for monitoring purposes and psychological support as well [30,31].

Smartphones. Smartphones (and other mobile devices such as tablets and smart watches) contribute to the monitoring scenario in a manifold fashion: they embed their own sensors, complementing wearable and environmental devices, and provide an accessible user interface, through which services can be made available to the end-users. Many apps exist, implementing relevant functions such as agenda, pill-reminder, physical activity tracker.

The monitoring scenario depicted so far features a quite varied set of devices, producing a large amount of heterogeneous data, which need to be fused and analysed by means of suitable data analytics techniques.

Analysis of smart home sensor data can be performed at different levels of abstraction. For example, especially for interaction sensors (e.g. toilet/fridge use), trends and anomalies can be detected effectively by adopting probabilistic framework and Bayesian analysis techniques [17]. In that case, it is possible to both detect interesting trends or anomalies, and, at the same time, express the confidence in such observation. Human behaviours are, indeed, extremely varied and noisy: estimating confidence in the predictions may help in significantly reduce false positives alarms. Trending analyses and anomaly detection can be combined at a higher level and correlations can be detected between different behaviours. Also, the combination of several behaviours may be used to explain others.

Another interesting application of smart home data analysis is the assessment of the inhabitant's functional abilities. For example, [12–14,32] mainly focus on recognizing ADLs or Instrumental ADL (IADL) to generate reports about the most common behaviours/activities of the subjects. Other works attempt to model the evolution of a suitably defined behaviour and aim at detecting anomalies or trends: for example, in [33,34], the use patterns of appliances are exploited to monitor the behaviour of an elderly resident and check whether it can be considered normal or anomalous. Instead, reference [35] model sequences of ADL, and check whether anomalies can be spotted, accounting for different time periods and days of the week, whereas [31] focuses on predicting the most likely next activity given the past ones. Machine learning techniques and probabilistic frameworks are commonly adopted to perform such analysis, e.g. by exploiting Hidden Markov Models (HMM) [36], Conditional Random Fields (CRF) [37], Support vector Machines (SVM) [32] and many others.

8.4 CARDEA AAL system

8.4.1 CARDEA architecture and main wireless sensors

In this section, a short description of the CARDEA System is given. CARDEA has been developed at Parma University, Italy, and has been deployed in many different installations context, such as private homes, residential facilities for the elderly, pilots projects of European AAL-JP (Ambient/Active Assisted Living – Joint Programme) [38].

CARDEA is composed of a set of networked wireless sensors and by a "gateway" node, that gathers sensor information and deals with the storage and communications of data. Among sensors, a wearable device has been developed (called MuSa) as well, which will be introduced in the next section. The wireless infrastructure of the CARDEA system exploit the IEEE 802.15.4/ZigBee communication protocol [39]. Besides standard devices (door/windows, PIR, etc.), some more application-specific sensors have been developed, aimed at providing relevant behavioural information, including:

Bed and Chair Occupancy Sensor. It consists of pressure-sensitive pads, connected to a wireless ZigBee Transmitter Module. Each time the user occupies or frees up the bed (or the chair), a message is sent over the ZigBee network. It provides information about sleeping patterns and daily habits, useful for behaviour profiling and for abnormal behavioural pattern recognition.

Fridge Sensor. It is a small box, to be placed inside the fridge, to provide some indirect information related to feeding habits. It detects door openings, and checks for internal temperature and humidity. Besides behavioural tracking, it also provide safety features, such as warnings if the door has been left open or the temperature exceeded the safe range.

Toilet Occupancy Sensor. Based on a proximity sensor, detects the actual toilet use and allows for checking frequency and counting visits: such parameters are relevant to many pathological scenarios indeed.

All wireless sensors communicate, by means of a ZigBee communication infrastructure, including a coordinator node and some routers, extending the network over an arbitrarily sized and shaped home environment. A central control unit, based on a keyboard- and monitor-less miniPC, supervises the network and allows for Internet connectivity. Such gateway (exploiting the Linux OS) also manages installation phases and continuously checks for sensor connectivity, collects and stores sensor data and forwards them to an upper level infrastructure (e.g. cloud-based storage and data analytics services).

8.4.2 The MuSA wearable sensor

Wearable sensors are a key component for monitoring human behaviour. The wireless sensor platform MuSA [40] (shown in Figure 8.1), which specifically targets the assistive context, has been designed and introduced in the CARDEA environment.

Internal MuSA architecture features a CC2531 SoC [41], which fully manages wireless communication as well as local data processing. MuSA embeds an Inertial Measurement Unit (IMU, ST device LSM9DS0-iNEM [42]), featuring a 3D digital linear acceleration sensor, a 3D digital angular rate sensor and a 3D digital magnetic sensor within the same chip. The IMU is exploited to evaluate human body position and orientation information, primarily aimed at fall detection purposes. Within the HELICOPTER scenario, MuSA is exploited for additional key functions: (i) estimating physical activity and (ii) supporting user identification and localization.

8.4.2.1 Physical activity estimation

Physical activity (PA) is a meaningful health indicator [43], which enters many "diagnostic suspicion" scenarios. To evaluate PA, some specific features of the motion pattern need to be identified: walking velocity is often regarded as an expressive indicator [44]. Accurate evaluation of the walking velocity, based on body-worn accelerometer, however, is a demanding task [45]. On the other hand, in the underpinned behavioural assessment, relative changes are mostly relevant to infer anomalies. In fact, referring to absolute velocity thresholds is unpractical: due to large variability in human behaviour, this would yield either too a coarse resolution in anomaly detection (suitable for detecting major safety issues only) or unacceptable false-alarm rates. We therefore selected a less overtaxing approach, by referring to

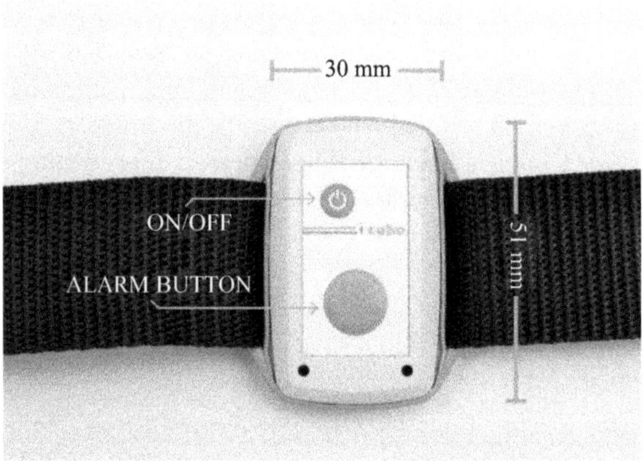

Figure 8.1 MuSA wearable device

the "energy expenditure" (EE) calculation introduced in [46]. According to such an approach, EE can be estimated by the simple relationship:

$$EE = k_1 + k_2 I_{A,tot}$$

where k_1 and k_2 are suitable constants (empirically characterized) and $I_{A,tot}$ depends on the acceleration components (a_x, a_y, a_z):

$$I_{A,tot} = \int_{TW} a_x dt + \int_{TW} a_y dt \int_{TW} a_z dt$$

Since each component is independently integrated over a short time window (TW), uncertainties related to noise and to integration drift error are minimized. The overall computation burden is therefore greatly reduced, allowing for implementing the algorithm in the MuSA firmware and thus enabling daylong monitoring.

The acceleration components (a_x, a_y, a_z) are sampled at a 60 Hz rate. Then a high-pass filter (Butterworth, fourth order) is applied, to eliminate frequency components at baseband and numerical integration is carried out. The radio-link is exploited to communicate synthesized EE data only, with no need of real-time transfer of large data streams, thus optimizing battery lifetime.

Despite its overall simplicity, such an approach still retains basic information about the intensity of physical activity, as shown in Figure 8.2. The figure reports the estimated EE for several (healthy) subjects walking on a motorized treadmill, the speed of which was incremented at 1 km/h/min intervals. A good repeatability of measurement is obtained across different subjects, and the ability of discriminating among different walking velocities and patterns is shown. In the example, when switching from 5 to 6 km/h, users started to run, thus exhibiting an abrupt increase in the EE value. Within the behavioural assessment scheme, EE is therefore assumed as both a quantitative (i.e. measuring PA intensity) and a qualitative indicator, by discriminating physically "active" and "inactive" periods during the daily activities.

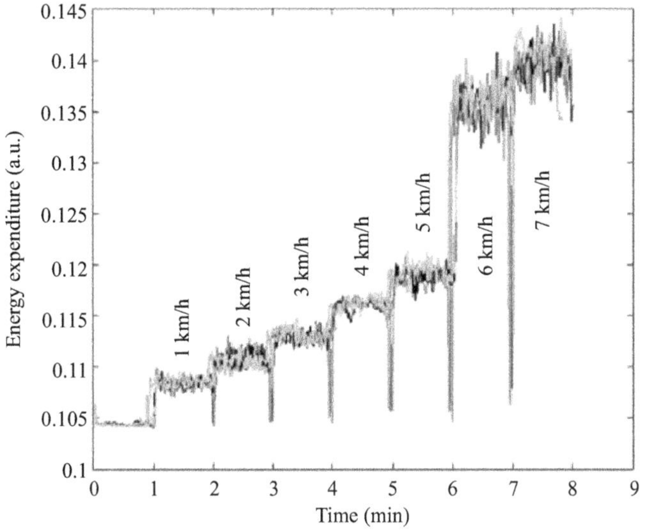

Figure 8.2 MuSA: on-board energy expenditure calculation

8.4.2.2 Localization and identification

As stated above, environmental devices can be used to assess the user behavioural profile: however, if more than one single person lives in the monitored environment, information coming from non-personal devices becomes not univocal: further qualifiers are needed to associate such information with the user actually performing the action. In principle, knowing the exact location of the user and of environmental devices in the home space would straightforwardly allow to perform such tagging. Indoor localization is a lively research field: many solutions have been proposed, based on various methods or technologies, ranging from RSSI [47] or time of flight [48] to geo-magnetic field [49] and Mutually Coupled Resonating Circuits [50].

In this case too, however, precise indoor localization can be regarded as an overkilling task, and a simpler, topological association may better match peculiar constraints on implementation intrusiveness and costs. We therefore adopt a proximity-based approach, which exploits wearable sensors (inherently carrying identification information) and native features of the radio communication protocols. In particular, the Received Signal Strength Index (RSSI) can be evaluated for every communication message; according to [51], RSSI can be correlated to the distance $d_{i,j}$ between a given transceiver couple (i,j):

$$d_{i,j} = k \cdot 10^{-RSSI_{i,j}}$$

where k is a constant involving signal propagation features, related to the actual signal path. Hence, a first tagging mechanism can be devised: every time an environmental sensor is activated, it polls all wearable devices within the home, and compares RSS indexes. The user wearing the device which features the highest RSSI (and thus the lower distance) is then identified as the one actually interacting. This does involve neither additional hardware components nor any prior knowledge about the sensor network and home physical features. It can therefore be regarded as a "plug & play" approach, requiring no home-specific calibration or training.

The above method relies on a few assumptions: first, the propagation constant k is assumed not to significantly vary among compared paths: while not holding in the general case, such assumption is reasonable when comparing path in the close nearby of the fixed-position environmental sensor. Second, the sensor activation is attributed to the closest user, which again seems to be acceptable in most real-life situation. Of course, propagation noise and crowded conditions may possibly limit accuracy: nevertheless, identification feature does not trigger any "mission-critical" activity and simply supports building of behavioural profiles, on a statistical basis. Hence, some errors possibly occurring in trickiest situations can be tolerated, just resulting in statistical noise and not jeopardizing the whole picture. Accuracy in the order of 90% was evaluated over a wide range of situations, in a multi-user, multiple-sensors lab emulating a living environment [52]. Sample identification data are reported in Figure 8.3, where data coming from environmental sensors are fused, according to the strategy described above, with wearable sensor data to provide identification. Gray data on the left refers to raw outputs of environmental sensors, while corresponding "tagged" data are reported on the right, along with EE estimates. Red ticks are marked when wearable sensors are inactive (thus preventing identification) or when the action is carried out by a third person (family member, caregivers). The approach can be generalized and strengthened by involving more devices in the identification

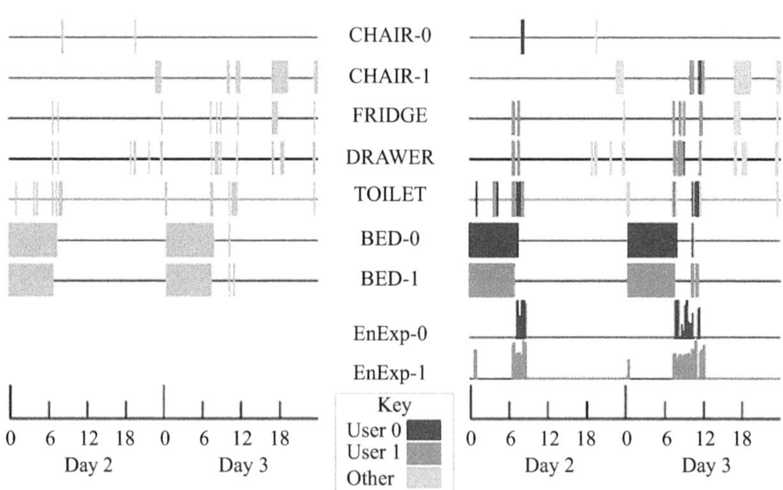

Figure 8.3 Tagged sensor activity data: environmental sensors only (left), EE calculation, sensor data tagging (right)

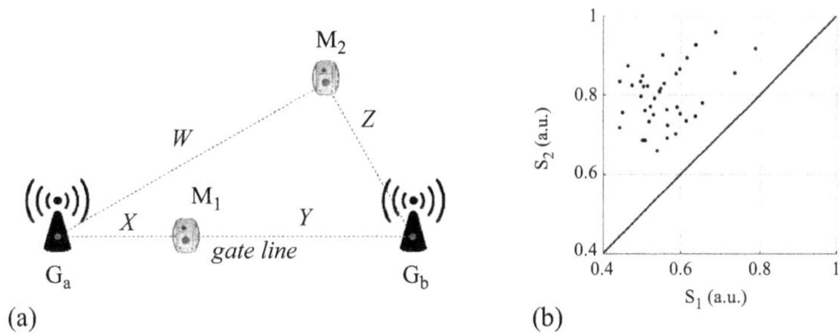

Figure 8.4 CARDEAgate approach. (a) Triangulation concept. (b) Distance sums scatter plot

procedure: Figure 8.4 illustrates the CARDEAgate concept, based on the interaction of wearable devices with a couple of radio-beacons placed at fixed positions. In this case, the transceivers themselves act as a sensor: whenever a person crosses the line between the beacons, the propagation features along such line are modified by the body absorption [53], this resulting in a consequent modulation of the RSS Index. CARDEAgate thus consists of a couple of ZigBee transceiver (Ga and Gb) each having the size of a standard USB flash drive. G_a and G_b exchange a message every 200 ms and monitor the RSSI: if a sudden loss is observed (i.e. the user's "shadow"), a person crossing the gateway is inferred.

Then, both G_a and G_b start independent, proximity-based identification procedures the results of which are fused at the supervision level. Elementary geometrical reasoning yields that the device crossing the gateway is the one that features the lowest sum of distances from either gate transceiver. In Figure 8.4, for instance, M_1 is the device crossing the gate line, whereas M_2 lies nearby (being possibly closer to either beacon than M_1). Thus:

$$x + y < w + z$$

where x, y, w and z are the distance between mobile and fixed nodes, as indicated in figure. We define the distance sum and obtain:

$$S_j = d_{j,A} + d_{j,B} = k(10^{-RSSI_{1,A}} + 10^{-RSSI_{1,B}})$$

so that, if the inequality $S_1 < S_2$ holds true, the crossing of M_1 is assessed, and M_2 otherwise. Such a test is straightforwardly generalizable to a larger number of involved users.

The approach has been validated on different test conditions, evaluating both detection (i.e. the ability of recognizing a person's passage) and identification performance [54]. A simple test is summarized in Figure 8.4 (right), referring to a two-user scenario, in which a person wearing a MuSA (M_1) walked through the gateway (installed on an actual door) and another person, wearing a second MuSA (M_2), was wandering around, in random positions. Around 40 tries were carried out and the results were evaluated, illustrated by the scatter plot in figure, where every point refer to the S_1 and S_2 estimation for a given condition. As shown, all conditions where correctly interpreted (i.e. $S_1 < S_2$), with the clearance from the diagonal line providing a confidence indicator for the inferred information.

8.4.3 CARDEA user interface

In the context of human monitoring for elderly care, different interfaces need to be devised, depending on the actual end-user involved. To the primary end-user (the elderly person himself) the UI should provide basic motivational information, and simple system status checks, reassuring him about proper functioning of the system. Secondary end-users (i.e. informal and formal caregivers) are instead much more involved in actual interaction: they do not necessarily have advanced technical skill, so that usability and accessibility are main concerns in this case too. The interface must be easy to read and immediately understandable; behavioural data must be illustrated in a simple, intuitive fashion. To this purpose, CARDEA features a web control panel, also suitable for visualization on mobile devices. Access is granted to users, according to different authorization levels, depending on the user's role in the care network. The main page plainly shows the state and of the CARDEA sensors network. Also some timing information are given in an intuitive format (Figure 8.5), which allows the caregiver to obtain, at a glance, an overall feeling of the current situation. Checking for abnormal conditions can be programmed, according to the actual needs, and may result in proper alarm signalling. For instance, a fall detection triggers the alarm signal shown in Figure 8.6. At the same time, phone calls and text messages

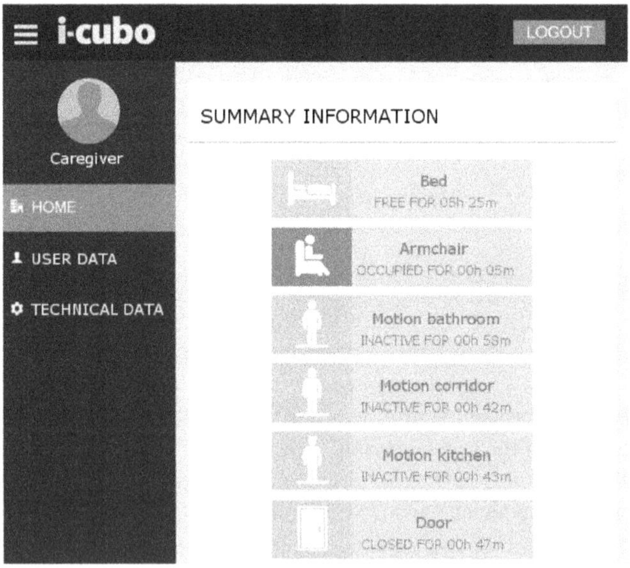

Figure 8.5 A screenshot of the main page of the CARDEA panel control

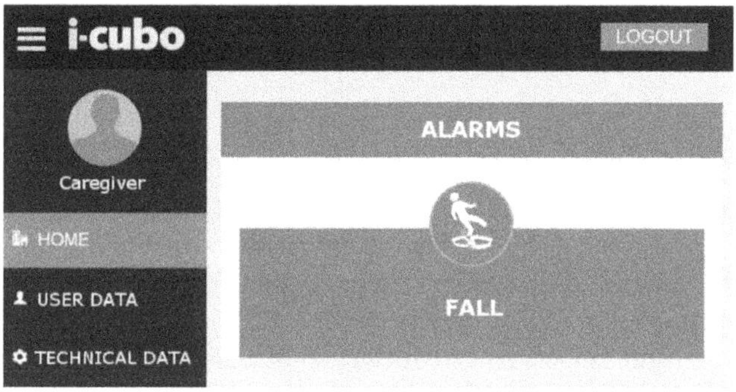

Figure 8.6 A screenshot of the main page of the CARDEA panel control – fall alarm message

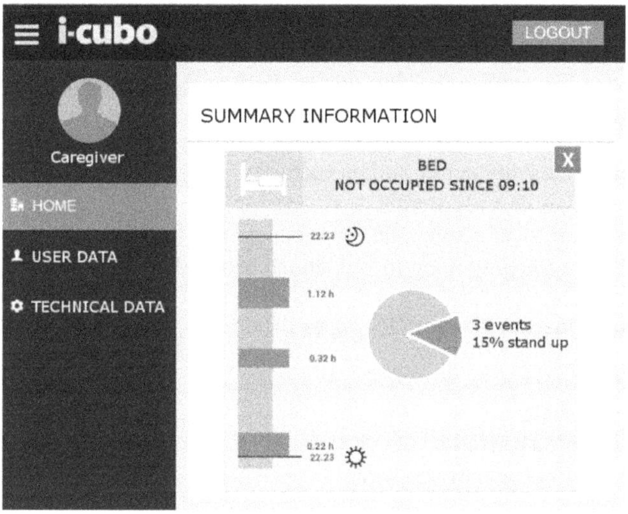

Figure 8.7 A screenshot of the main page of the CARDEA panel control – statistics information

can be programmed to reach relevant persons in the care network. Further insight can be gained by looking at usage statistics and trends measurements: in Figure 8.7, a sample of statics related to the bed occupancy is shown.

8.5 A case study: the helicopter AAL project

The HELICOPTER [55] project, carried out in the framework of the European AAL Joint Programme, aims at implementing strategies for prevention and early discovery of age-related diseases by means of effective interaction among environmental and clinical sensing technologies [55]. In the following, the project scope and service implementation will be presented, along with the results.

8.5.1 HELICOPTER service concept

Many chronic diseases, endemic among elderly population, could be more effectively treated (or even prevented) by accounting for frequent monitoring of suitable indicators. As stated in the introduction, a more comprehensive view can be achieved by complementing telemedicine services with AAL components, providing indirect health indicators and supporting early detection of anomalies. In the HELICOPTER view, a set of such anomalies may result in what we call a "diagnostic suspicion" and may address the user, or the caregivers, towards more accurate assessment, based on clinical evaluation.

In order to illustrate the system aim, we refer here to a simple example, related to the heart failure diagnostic suspicion. Congestive heart failure (CHF) is among the primary causes of hospitalization in elderly population, and regular lifestyle monitoring is recommended to control it and minimize its impact on quality of life. People suffering from CHF tend to develop one or more among the following behavioural indicators:

- Increased urinary frequency and/or nocturnal
- Sudden changes of body weight
- Decrease of physical activity, due to tiredness and fatigue
- Discomfort in sleeping lying in bed, due to oedema

Such indicators, in turn, can be detected by means of "not clinical" sensors:

- Toilet sensor
- Bodyweight scale
- Wearable motion sensor
- Bed and chair occupancy sensors

An inference engine combines outcomes of different home sensors and evaluates the likeliness of the heart failure condition. Once a possible CHF crisis is inferred, the user may be asked to self-check relevant physiological parameters by using networked clinical devices. In the example at hand, these include blood pressure and oxygen blood concentration measurement, which are then fed back to the behavioural model, to confirm or reject the diagnostic suspicion.

Similarly, a set of age-related diseases has been selected in the current HELICOPTER development stage, shaping related behavioural models. The model list includes:

- Hypoglycaemia
- Hyperglycaemia
- Cystitis
- Heart failure

- Depression
- Reduced physical autonomy
- Prostatic hypertrophy
- Bladder prolapse

Although each model may actually involve a different set of sensors, the overall hierarchy is similar, exploiting the environmental and wearable sensors for inferring potentially troublesome situations, to be confirmed by involving clinical devices into the evaluation.

The HELICOPTER service consists in the continuous scan of the overall sensors picture, aimed at early detection of "diagnostic suspicions": this would help the caregivers in better and earlier assessment of professional care needs, and provide the end-user with an increased safety feeling, coming from the awareness of being continuously watched over.

8.5.2 HELICOPTER system architecture

The system architecture exploits a heterogeneous layer of sensing devices, which includes:

- Clinical sensors, which provide the system with accurate data about physiological parameters, implying user awareness and collaboration. In the current implementation, a bodyweight scale, a blood pressure monitor, a pulsoxymeter and a glucose meter have been included. Commercial, off-the-shelf devices have been selected, the overall system being open to further addition or different suppliers.
- Environmental sensors, providing data related to the user interaction with the home environment, linked to behavioural meaningful patterns. This includes: room presence sensors, bed or chair occupancy sensors, fridge and cupboard sensors (to monitor feeding habits), toilet sensors, power meters (to monitor appliances usage; e.g. TV set). In this case, no user awareness or activation is required.
- Wearable devices, which provide information about individual physical activity, also enabling emergency button services.

All sensors are seamlessly connected in a virtual network: however, different wireless protocols are exploited at the physical level. Namely, clinical sensors exploit standard Bluetooth communication technology, following telemedicine mainstream technologies, whereas environmental and wearable sensors exploits the ZigBee communication protocol, in compliance with the "Home automation" ZigBee profiles [56].

Data coming from all the wireless sensors are gathered by a home gateway device, consisting of a tiny/embedded PC, which runs a supervision process and takes care of data storage. Data coming from the peripheral devices are abstracted, making them independent of the actual physical feature of the given sensor. The HELICOPTER database enables communication among different system modules: in particular, behavioural analysis and anomaly detection are carried out by dedicated modules, periodically querying the database. Similarly, a variety of interfaces can be implemented (aimed at end-users or caregivers) which exploit the database contents for providing appropriate feedbacks. That is, the database is at the crossroads among different subsystems (sensing, processing, interfaces) and thus supports system modularity; a suitable data structure has been devised and implemented, exploiting a MySQL open-source architecture.

8.5.3 Results

The HELICOPTER system is being tested within a living-lab approach, availing itself of nearly 35 pilot homes implemented in the Netherlands and in Sweden. About 50 (65+) end-users are involved, both living alone or in couples.

In Figure 8.8 data coming from environmental sensors are shown, as sampled for a week period in a dwelling where a couple lives. The identification strategy allows for effectively tagging most of the sensor data, allowing to build the knowledge base upon which anomaly detection can be carried out.

Consistent views of user's daily life routines can be gained from such a plot. For instance, quite different users' sleeping patterns can be appreciated.

In Figure 8.9, a "heatmap" showing average distribution of sensors events along the daytime is shown, making such a difference more clearly visible.

It is self-evident that such data include valuable information: the key issue here is to make such information perceivable by caregivers in a straightforward fashion, without requiring to analyse too complex technical visualizations and possibly introducing some automatic flagging mechanisms, based on machine learning and artificial reasoning.

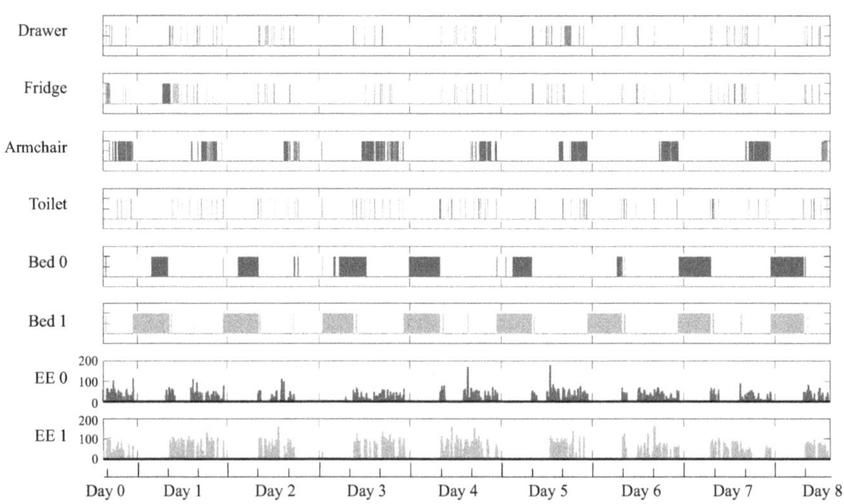

Figure 8.8 Activity log from the HELICOPTER sensor network (NL_01 pilot, 2 persons)

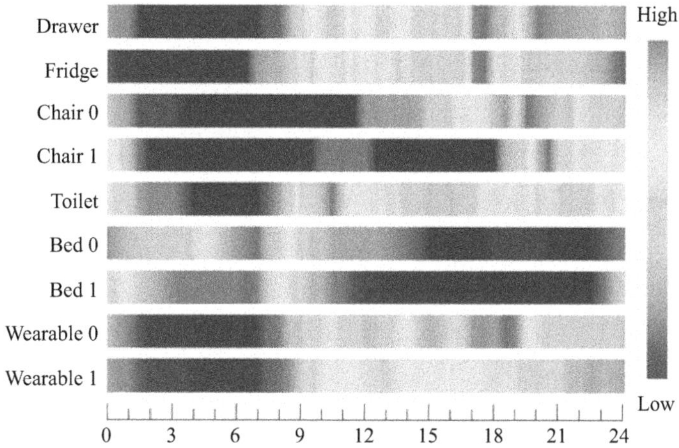

Figure 8.9 Normalized average activity profiles for environmental sensors (NL_01 pilot, 2 persons)

For instance, from gathered data it is possible to extract the so-called activity curves. Such curves attempt to model the distribution of the mean percentage of time that a sensor is active within a given time slot. In order to derive such distributions, the data are first grouped by specific time slots (e.g. 30 min bins); then, using a bootstrapping procedure, the distribution of the mean is estimated, along with confidence intervals. Bootstrapping is performed to achieve a more robust estimation of the confidence intervals, since such analyses can be restricted to a few weeks, thus reducing the sample size. The choice of the binning size plays an important role too in the analysis of such data: setting too long windows may lead to a suppression of relevant behavioural information, whereas too short windows may yield noisy estimates. Figure 8.10 shows an example of such curves for a bed (a) and chair (b) sensor of a single-resident pilot; resolution of the time slots is set to 30 min. Each plot features two curves, belonging to different periods (in this case April vs. May). Statistical hypothesis testing via permutation tests is then performed, to assess whether there are significant deviations between the two different periods at each time bin. The resulting p-values are adjusted using the Holm–Bonferroni procedure, in order to account for multiple comparisons; the resulting statistically significant differences are then flagged by the system. In Figure 10(b), for example, a significant difference at 17:00 is detected for the armchair sensor ($p < 0.01$).

That is, by comparing profiles and related confidence intervals, the system is able to automatically rise an "attention" flag whenever a meaningful (abnormal) event occurs. Such detection actually adapts itself to the given user actual behaviour and is therefore suitable for deployment at different context, with no need of parameters specific tuning, with the system "calibration" occurring automatically and continuously throughout the system running time.

Another possible analysis technique aims at detecting trend and anomalies in count or percent of "active" data. Figure 8.11 shows such an example, with reference to

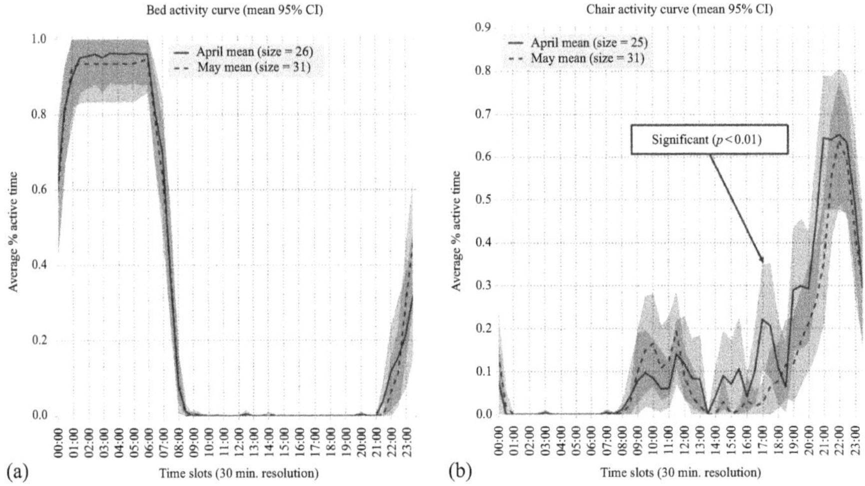

Figure 8.10 Activity curves from the HELICOPTER sensor network (NL_14 pilot, 1 person). (a) Bed sensor mean (and 95% CI) percent active time. (b) Chair sensor mean (and 95% CI) percent active time

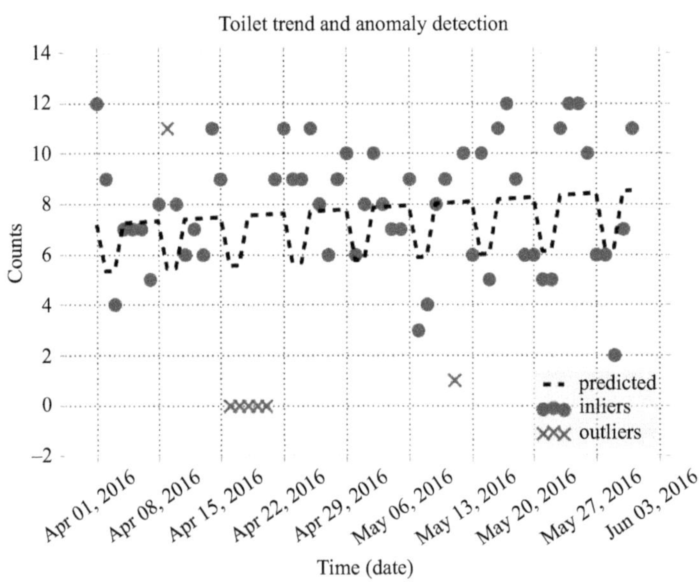

Figure 8.11 Trend and anomaly detection on toilet sensor event data (NL_14 pilot, 1 person). The black solid line is the predicted average counts, whereas outliers are flagged as red dots in the scatter plot

the toilet sensor. For discrete count data, a pre-processing step is applied: in fact, presence sensors (such as the toilet sensor) may fire repeatedly despite a single "activity" being detected. Raw data are thus aggregated to estimate the number of independent events, and this value is used to carry on further investigations. Without any loss of generality, let us consider the independent toilet visits throughout the day. Gross outliers are initially flagged; then, the count data are fed into a robust Poisson regression module, which attempts to explain the expected number of toilet visits using the following features:

- bias term: the overall average number of visits
- linear trend term: a linearly increasing feature trying to detect longitudinal increments (or decreases)
- week-day vs. week-end day: a feature which allows to have different behaviour between week-days and weekends

The model fitting allows to estimate the impact of each feature, which is a useful behavioural indicator. Furthermore, outliers which deviate too much from the model are detected and flagged, as shown in Figure 8.11 (crosses). As in the previous example, thus, the caregiver may get a simple anomaly "flag" information, automatically worked out by the system, without necessarily having to cope with more complex data visualization or analysis tool.

8.6 Conclusions

In this chapter, an account of human monitoring technologies exploiting ambient assisted living environments is given. Of course, the field is too wide and dynamic to lend itself to an exhaustive discussion; the main outcomes of the above discussion may therefore be summarized as follows:

- Ambient assisted living and smart home paradigms inherently provide much data which are suitable for tracking human behaviours, this possibly providing relevant insights about user's health and its evolution in time.
- Based on the indirect clues coming from behavioural analysis, "indirect" monitoring approaches can be devised, featuring less intrusive and more continuous features with respect, for instance, to telemedicine approach. By combining such complementary views, a more effective and comprehensive monitoring tool can be obtained.
- To deal with the resulting, highly heterogeneous, sensing infrastructure, smart analysis techniques are needed, to fuse data and to infer from them information meaningful to caregivers, in a format readily understandable and not requiring specific technical skill for its interpretation.
- As an example, the CARDEA monitoring environment has been discussed, highlighting some specific features suitable for assistive purposes. In particular, environmental and wearable devices, straightforwardly producing behaviourally meaningful data have been presented.

- Hints about data analytics techniques, based on machine learning and suitable for dealing with the large variability of human behaviour and needs have been introduced.

In conclusion, on the one hand human monitoring obviously represents an inherent potential outcome of the imminent IoT scenario; on the other hand, however, dealing with elderly persons and with their supporting network involves a number of design constraints, coming from usability, accessibility and ethical concerns, which needs to be take into account in every phase of technology design.

References

[1] "People in the EU – who are we and how do we live?" EUROSTAT website, available from http://ec.europa.eu/eurostat/en/web/products-statistical-books/-/KS-04-15-567 [Last accessed 25/01/2017].

[2] "People in the EU – population projections", EUROSTAT website, available from http://ec.europa.eu/eurostat/statistics-explained/index.php/People_in_the_EU_%E2%80%93_population_projections [Last accessed 25/01/2017].

[3] "Ageing and welfare state policies", Economic and Financial Affairs section of European Commission website, available from http://ec.europa.eu/economy_finance/structural_reforms/ageing/index_en.htm [Last accessed 25/01/2017].

[4] Losardo A., Bianchi V., Grossi F., Matrella G., De Munari I. and Ciampolini P., "Web-enabled home assistive tools", *Assistive Technology Research Series*, vol. 29, pp. 448–455, 2011.

[5] Losardo A., Grossi F., Matrella G., De Munari I. and Ciampolini P., "Exploiting AAL environment for behavioral analysis", *Assistive Technology Research Series*, vol. 33, pp. 1121–1125, 2013.

[6] HELICOPTER AAL-JP Project Official website, available from http://www.helicopter-aal.eu/ [Last accessed 25/01/2017].

[7] Mao R., Xu H., Wu W., Li J., Li Y. and Lu M., "Overcoming the challenge of variety: big data abstraction, the next evolution of data management for AAL communication systems", *IEEE Communications Magazine*, vol. 53, no. 1, pp. 42–47, January 2015.

[8] Cunha D., Trevisan G., Samagaio F., *et al.* "Ambient assisted living technology: comparative perspectives of users and caregivers", *2013 IEEE 15th International Conference on e-Health Networking, Applications & Services (Healthcom)*, Lisbon, 2013, pp. 41–45.

[9] Rashidi P. and Mihailidis A., "A survey on ambient-assisted living tools for older adults", *IEEE Journal of Biomedical and Health Informatics*, vol. 17, no. 3, pp. 579–590, May 2013.

[10] Geman O., Sanei S., Costin H.-N., *et al.* "Challenges and trends in ambient assisted living and intelligent tools for disabled and elderly people",

2015 International Workshop on Computational Intelligence for Multimedia Understanding (IWCIM), Prague, 2015, pp. 1–5.

[11] Galarraga M., Serrano L., Martinez I., De Toledo P. and Reynolds M., "Telemonitoring systems interoperability challenge: an updated review of the applicability of ISO/IEEE 11073 Standards for Interoperability in Telemonitoring", *29th Annual International Conference of the IEEE Engineering in Medicine and Biology Society*, Lyon, 2007, pp. 6161–6165.

[12] Cook D.J., "Learning setting-generalized activity models for smart spaces", *IEEE Intelligent Systems*, vol. 27, no. 1, pp. 32–38, 2012.

[13] De Silva L.C., Chamin M. and Iskandar M.P., "State of the art of smart homes", *Engineering Applications of Artificial Intelligence*, vol. 25, no. 7, pp. 1313–1321, 2012.

[14] Das S.J. and Cook D.J., "Designing smart environments: a paradigm based on learning and prediction", *Proceedings of the International Conference on Pattern Recognition and Machine Intelligence (PReMI-LNCS)*, Kolkata, India, 2005, pp. 80–90.

[15] Guerra C., Montalto F., Bianchi V., De Munari I. and Ciampolini P., "A low-cost zigbee-based gateway system for indoor localization and identification of a person", *Lecture Notes in Computer Science (including subseries Lecture Notes in Artificial Intelligence and Lecture Notes in Bioinformatics)*, vol. 8868, pp. 179–186, 2014.

[16] Guerra C., Bianchi V., De Munari I. and Ciampolini P., "An identification procedure for behavioral analysis in a multi-user environment", *Studies in Health Technology and Informatics*, vol. 217, pp. 282–287, 2015.

[17] Mora N., Losardo A., De Munari I. and Ciampolini P., "Self-tuning behavioral analysis in AAL FOOD project pilot environments", *Studies in Health Technology and Informatics*, vol. 217, pp. 295–299, 2015.

[18] Vespasiani G., Corradetti I., Pierantozzi N., *et al.*, "AALISABETH: home environment cooperating to health assessment", *Gerontechnology*, vol. 13, no. 2, p. 293, 2014.

[19] Grossi F., Bianchi V., Matrella G., De Munari I. and Ciampolini P., "Senior-friendly kitchen activity: the FOOD Project", *Gerontechnology*, vol. 13, no. 2, p. 200, 2014.

[20] Burzagli L., Di Fonzo L., Emiliani P.L., *et al.*, "The FOOD project: interacting with distributed intelligence in the kitchen environment", *Lecture Notes in Computer Science (including subseries Lecture Notes in Artificial Intelligence and Lecture Notes in Bioinformatics)*, Lecture Notes in Computer Science, vol. 8515 (PART 3), pp. 463–474, 2014.

[21] Allen J., Boffi L., Burzagli L., Ciampolini P., De Munari I. and Emiliani P.L., "FOOD: discovering techno-social scenarios for networked kitchen systems", *Assistive Technology Research Series*, vol. 33, pp. 143–1148, 2013.

[22] Matrella G., Grossi F., Bianchi V., De Munari I. and Ciampolini P., "An environmental control HW/SW framework for daily living of elderly and disabled people", *Proceedings of the Fourth IASTED International Conference on Telehealth and Assistive Technologies*, Baltimore, MD, pp. 87–92, 2008.

[23] Grossi F., Matrella G., De Munari I. and Ciampolini P., “A flexible home automation system applied to elderly care”, *Digest of Technical Papers – IEEE International Conference on Consumer Electronics*, 2007.
[24] Bianchi V., Grossi F., De Munari I. and Ciampolini P., “Integrating fall detection into a home control system”, *Assistive Technology Research Series*, vol. 25, pp. 322–326, 2009.
[25] Wan J., Byrne C.A., O’Grady M.J. and O’Hare G.M.P., “Managing wandering risk in people with dementia”, *IEEE Transactions on Human–Machine Systems*, vol. 45, no. 6, pp. 819–823, Dec. 2015.
[26] Grossi F., Bianchi V., Matrella G., De Munari I. and Ciampolini P., “Internet-based home monitoring and control”, *Assistive Technology Research Series*, vol. 25, pp. 309–313, 2009.
[27] Ciampolini P., De Munari I., Matrella G., Grossi F. and Bianchi V., “An ‘assistance over IP’ network for monitoring and support of daily living activities”, *Assistive Technology Research Series*, vol. 20, pp. 743–747, 2007.
[28] Bianchi V., Guerra C., De Munari I. and Ciampolini P., “A wearable sensor for AAL-based continuous monitoring”, *Lecture Notes in Computer Science (including subseries Lecture Notes in Artificial Intelligence and Lecture Notes in Bioinformatics)*, vol. 9677, pp. 383–394, 2016.
[29] Montalto F., Bianchi V., De Munari I. and Ciampolini P., “A wearable assistive device for AAL applications”, *Assistive Technology Research Series*, vol. 33, pp. 101–106, 2013.
[30] Manti M., Pratesi A., Falotico E., Cianchetti M. and Laschi C., “Soft assistive robot for personal care of elderly people”, *Sixth IEEE International Conference on Biomedical Robotics and Biomechatronics (BioRob)*, Singapore, 2016, pp. 833–838.
[31] Yang L., Song X., Li Y., Shan H. and Guo J., “Design and experimental research on intelligent household assistive robot for the elderly”, *Fifth International Conference on Instrumentation and Measurement, Computer, Communication and Control (IMCCC)*, Qinhuangdao, 2015, pp. 1316–1319.
[32] Cook D.J., Crandall A.S., Thomas B.L. and Krishnan N.C., “CASAS: a smart home in a box”, *Computer*, vol. 46, no. 7, pp. 62–69, 2013.
[33] Suryadevara N.K., Mukhopadhyay S.C., Wang R. and Rayudu R.K., “Forecasting the behavior of an elderly using wireless sensors data in a smart home”, *Engineering Applications of Artificial Intelligence*, vol. 26, no. 10, pp. 2641–2652, 2013.
[34] Suryadevara N.K., Gaddam A., Rayudu R.K. and Mukhopadhyay S.C., “Wireless sensors network based safe home to care elderly people: behaviour detection”, *Sensors and Actuators A: Physical*, vol. 186, pp. 277–283, 2012.
[35] Hoque E., Dickerson R.F., Preum S.M., Hanson M., Barth A. and Stankovic J.A., “Holmes: a comprehensive anomaly detection system for daily in-home activities”, *International Conference on Distributed Computing in Sensor Systems*, Fortaleza, Brazil, 2015, pp. 40–51.
[36] Cook D.J., “Learning setting-generalized activity models for smart spaces”, *IEEE Intelligent Systems*, vol. 27, no. 1, pp. 32–38, 2012.

[37] Nazerfard E., Das B., Holder L.B. and Cook D.J., "Conditional random fields for activity recognition in smart environments", *Proceedings of the First ACM International Health Informatics Symposium*, Arlington, VA, 2010, pp. 282–286.
[38] "AAL Programme, Active and Assisted Living Programme – ICT for ageing well" website, available from http://www.aal-europe.eu/ [Last accessed 25/01/2017].
[39] Bianchi V., Grossi F., Matrella G., De Munari I. and Ciampolini P., "A wireless sensor platform for assistive technology applications", *Proceedings of the 11th EUROMICRO Conference on Digital System Design Architectures, Methods and Tools*, Parma, Italy, January, pp. 809–816, 2008.
[40] Bianchi V., Grossi F., De Munari I. and Ciampolini P., "MuSA: a multisensor wearable device for AAL", *Federated Conference on Computer Science and Information Systems (FedCSIS)*, Szczecin, Poland, 2011, pp. 375–380.
[41] http://www.ti.com/product/cc2531 [Last accessed: 26/01/2017].
[42] http://www.st.com/en/mems-and-sensors/lsm9ds0.html – product description [Last accessed: 26/01/2017].
[43] Montalto F., Bianchi V., De Munari I. and Ciampolini P., "Detection of elderly activity by the wearable sensor MuSA", *Gerontechnology*, vol. 13, no. 2, p. 264, 2014.
[44] Studenski S., Perera S., Patel K., *et al.* "Gait speed and survival in older adults", *Journal of the American Medical Association*, vol. 305, no. 1, pp. 50–58, 2011.
[45] Yang S. and Li Q., "Inertial sensor-based methods in walking speed estimation: a systematic review", *Sensors (Switzerland)*, vol. 12, no. 5, pp. 6102–6116, 2012.
[46] Bouten C.V., Westerterp K.R., Verduin M. and Janssen J.D., "Assessment of energy expenditure for physical activity using a triaxial accelerometer", *Medicine & Science in Sports & Exercise*, vol. 26, no. 12, pp. 1516–1523, 1995.
[47] Tian Y., Denby B., Ahriz I. and Roussel P., "Practical indoor localization using ambient RF", *IEEE Instrumentation and Measurement Technology Conference*, Minneapolis, MN, Minneapolis, MN, 2013, pp. 1125–1129.
[48] Santinelli G., Giglietti R. and Moschitta A., "Self-calibrating indoor positioning system based on ZigBee devices", *IEEE International Instrumentation and Measurement Conference*, Singapore, Singapore, pp. 1205–1210, 2009.
[49] Saxena A. and Zawodniok M., "Indoor positioning system using geo-magnetic field", *IEEE Instrumentation and Measurement Technology Conference*, Montevideo, Uruguay, pp. 572–577, 2014.
[50] De Angelis G., De Angelis A., Dionigi M., Mongiardo M., Moschitta A. and Carbone P., "An accurate indoor positioning-measurement system using mutually coupled resonating circuits", *IEEE International Instrumentation and Measurement Technology Conference (I2MTC) Proceedings*, Montevideo, Uruguay, pp. 844–849, 2014.

[51] Wilson J. and Patwari N., "Radio tomographic imaging with wireless networks", *IEEE Transactions on Mobile Computing*, vol. 9, no. 5, pp. 621–632, 2010.

[52] Guerra C., Bianchi V., De Munari I. and Ciampolini P., "Action tagging in a multi-user indoor environment for behavioural analysis purposes", *Proceedings of the Annual International Conference of the IEEE Engineering in Medicine and Biology Society (EMBS)*, Milan, Italy, 2015, November, pp. 5036–5039.

[53] Halder S.J., Park J.G., and Kim W. "Adaptive filtering for indoor localization using ZIGBEE RSSI and LQI measurement, Adaptive Filtering Applications", Dr Lino Garcia (Ed.), InTech, pp. 305–324, 2011. DOI: 10.5772/16441. Available from: https://www.intechopen.com/books/adaptive-filtering-applications/adaptive-filtering-for-indoor-localization-using-zigbee-rssi-and-lqi-measurement.

[54] Guerra C., Bianchi V., De Munari I. and Ciampolini P., "CARDEAGate: low-cost, ZigBee-based localization and identification for AAL purposes", *IEEE Instrumentation and Measurement Technology Conference*, Pisa, Italy, 2015, July, pp. 245–249.

[55] Guerra C., Bianchi V., Grossi F., *et al.*, "The HELICOPTER project: a heterogeneous sensor network suitable for behavioral monitoring", *Lecture Notes in Computer Science (including subseries Lecture Notes in Artificial Intelligence and Lecture Notes in Bioinformatics)*, 2015, vol. 9455, pp. 152–163.

[56] http://www.zigbee.org – ZigBee Alliance web site [Last accessed: 26/01/2017].

Chapter 9

Ambient intelligence for health: advances in vital signs and gait monitoring systems within mHealth environments

Jesús Fontecha, Iván Gónzalez, Vladimir Villarreal, and José Bravo

Abstract

This chapter presents an overview about the application of Ambient Intelligence to Healthcare environments, and how the current use of mobile devices provides new opportunities and determines new research areas such as mHealth, focused on the use of mobile technologies to improve people quality life getting clinical benefits. In this sense, monitoring is an important branch today in which researchers are working. There are many systems to monitor several factors regarding health.

In our case, three kinds of monitoring systems are detailed. The first approach describes a framework-based system to monitor several diseases like diabetes taking into account the most common factors. In the second case, we present the importance of long-term gait monitoring to detect frailty symptoms in early stages by developing software system and hardware infrastructures based on a variety of sensors. Finally, we detail an analysis tool to measure the level of performance of Instrumental Activities of Daily Living (IADL) of elderly people at home. Likewise, this tool provides some functionalities to assess level stress and quality of life of caregivers by conducting questionnaires.

Besides the description of the systems, we detail the evaluations carried out in each. We show the results according to system characteristics, usability, functionality and deployment of features among others.

9.1 Introduction

Birth of Ambient Intelligence (AmI) and Ubiquitous Computing paradigms meant a change in development and deployment of technological solutions capable of providing services adapted to the user and the environment [1]. The emergence of new technologies and smart devices helps us to improve different aspects of everyday life. In Health domain, there is an increase in the use of information systems by clinicians and patients. Mobile computing and wireless communication facilitate the development of applications to deal with numerous diseases and pathologies. In this sense, the use of mobile technologies and systems in health environments leads to a new concept known as mHealth. Most of mHealth works are focused on monitoring relevant parameters and diseases from individuals. Currently, there are monitoring devices that they are used by people to monitor physical activity, sleep and heart rate among others. However, a specific monitoring according to clinical purposes would provide real benefits in patients with chronic and non-chronic diseases and even to analyse parameters from everyday activities to improve their quality of life. In this chapter, we present a detailed overview about the concept of AmI-Health, and how Mobile Computing is changing the scenario of information systems in health environments. Thus, we study the application of Mobile Computing in health domain (mHealth), creating ecosystems that provide help and assistance to patients and clinicians in monitoring tasks. Besides, three kinds of systems related to health monitoring tasks have been developed and evaluated, showing the most outstanding experiences about these.

Section 9.2 shows the inclusion of Health systems under the Ambient Intelligent perspective and its evolution to mHealth. In Section 9.3, we detail the most common ecosystems and scenarios of mHealth solutions, and the importance of mobile monitoring (Section 9.3.1). Section 9.4 details three different systems developed to monitor vital signs, gait and everyday activities of people. Also, evaluation and results are presented. Finally, Section 9.5 shows the conclusions of this chapter.

9.2 From ambient intelligence to mHealth

AmI can be defined as the combination of Ubiquitous Computing, Natural Interfaces and Ubiquitous Communications to provide services in the environment according to user needs [2,3]. Nijholt [4] said "Ambient Intelligence consists of Ubiquitous Computing + intelligent and social interfaces which allow social interaction". In this sense, the search of new simple and natural ways of user interaction with computational devices in a specific environment has been the main research line from AmI paradigm. The emergence of smart and embedded technologies facilitates the application of this approach. When the principles of AmI [5] are applied to health environments a new research line known as AmIHealth (Ambient Intelligent for Health) arises, considering mobile devices an essential system for providing ubiquitous services to users.

Mobile Computing is a branch of Computer Science in which different devices and hardware systems are able to work and transmit information without being physically connected to a network. The main features of Mobile Computing include: mobility, far-reaching, ubiquity, convenience, instant connectivity, personalisation and localisation [6]. Currently, health domain is a key area to integrate mobile technologies, improving procedures regarding telemedicine, patient monitoring, location services, smart emergency response and access to patient records among others [7].

The term of mHealth is defined as the application of Mobile Computing in health domain using smartphones, tablets, monitoring devices and other wireless systems.

mHealth is a recent field that comes from e-Healthcare [8] whose aim was focused on providing technological and healthcare services in underdeveloped countries. Wireless capabilities of these systems allow us to gather health information with no physical connection between devices among other advantages [9]. Thus, patients and medical staff can get and provide services by using their mobile devices.

High growth in the use of Smartphones make them the most widespread electronic device in the world. In fact, by 2018 there will be 10 billion of Smartphones, more than the number of inhabitants. Their small size, process, storage and communication capabilities are speeding up deployment of systems and applications, especially in mHealth area. Furthermore, embedding sensors into Smartphones enable new possibilities to be used in health environments [10–12].

Before the mHealth term came into being, the concept of "unwired e-med" was introduced as a movement from telemedicine to wireless and mobile Internet applications [13]. Subsequently, wireless communications, networks and wearable systems have advanced significantly [14,15]. These improvements have had a substantial impact on e-Health. The benefits of wireless technology have been illustrated in the literature [16]. Using this technology, information about patients is easily accessible to clinicians, independently of their location. Traditionally, wireless solutions in healthcare are associated with "biomonitoring" by including parameters such as heart rate, blood pressure, blood oximetry and other vital signs. Other areas include movement monitoring, such as fall detection, physical activities, location tracking, and gait analysis.

Nowadays, the wide use of mobile systems facilitates the deployment of AmI-Health solutions. Building ecosystems where patients and clinical staff can get services adapted to their needs is a very important part of mHealth and SmartHealth paradigms.

9.3 mHealth

mHealth means Mobile Health and it is defined as a "medical and public health practise supported by mobile devices, such as mobile phones, patient monitoring devices, personal digital assistants (PDAs), and other wireless devices" [8]. Others define mHealth as "emerging mobile communication and network technologies for healthcare systems" [12]. More recently, the Foundation for the National Institutes for Health (FNIH) defined mHealth as "the delivery of healthcare services via mobile communication devices". It is intended to be a complement in healthcare tasks of doctors and clinicians where smart and mobile devices support their everyday tasks, even make easier the self-control of their own patients.

All mHealth systems should meet the following features determined by the FNIH: use of smart and mobile devices, inclusion of wireless technology and easy social adoption. Likewise, the main goals of mHealth solutions include: better management of health, make better healthcare decisions, find appropriate care, engage people and access providers, and management of ongoing health (monitoring).

The steady growth of mobile devices in the population, as well as the increase of their capabilities, enable us to perform healthcare tasks in everyday life. Last research works propose an evolution of mHealth concept to Smart Health [17], being an important branch in the development of future Smart cities.

According to the literature, we identify two key areas to deploy mHealth solutions: wellbeing in ageing and diseases (chronic and non-chronic) monitoring. In the first case, people live longer, with the estimation that there will be about 1.5 billion people aged more than 65 by 2050 [18]. The impact of this demographic change represents a challenge for governments and researchers worldwide, and new research lines have been created to deal with this. Ambient Assisted Living (AAL) aims to create healthcare systems to promote wellbeing in elderly people who live at home.

Monitoring of chronic and non-chronic diseases can be addressed with new technologies and mobile devices based on mHealth approaches. In fact, most mHealth systems are focused on monitoring tasks, in which results can be studied and analysed by other systems as well as by doctors and researchers. In the next section, we are going to explain the importance of monitoring in more detail.

Currently, mHealth system is a small piece of a more complex system known as ecosystem. In nature, ecosystem is defined as "a community of living organisms in conjunction with the nonliving components of their environments (things like air, water and mineral soil), interacting as a system" [19]. However, there is not a standard definition for mHealth ecosystem in the literature. Similarly, we can define this as "a community of people who interact with mobile devices of an environment to get clinical benefits".

All mHealth systems should take into account an appropriate relationship between technology and the following: users, mobile devices, data, connectivity and sensors. The consistency of mHealth solutions should remain although we have different kinds of users, different mobile systems, several mechanisms of data acquisition and storage and a variety of sensors.

Furthermore, the use of smart devices such as activity bracelets, wearable devices, smartwatches and the own smartphones in our society can be exploited to monitor a large number of diseases and pathologies as an important part of mHealth systems.

9.3.1 Mobile monitoring

One of the most important areas in development of mHealth systems refers to monitoring. Current technologies and communication capabilities allow us to gather relevant data about patients or simple users as well as to provide the mechanisms for analysing such information [20].

There are many systems dedicated to monitor several parameters or activities of users facilitating self-control or a control by other users such as relatives or clinicians. Almost all monitoring proposals share some elements and actions. Figure 9.1 represents a common scenario of mobile monitoring system, in this case to perform monitoring of obese patients. Thus, we have four groups of identified elements: users, environments, sensors and devices, and communication technologies. The information flows are given between computational devices associated with users and environments. Each device has one or more objectives regarding monitoring, data visualisation or analysis of information.

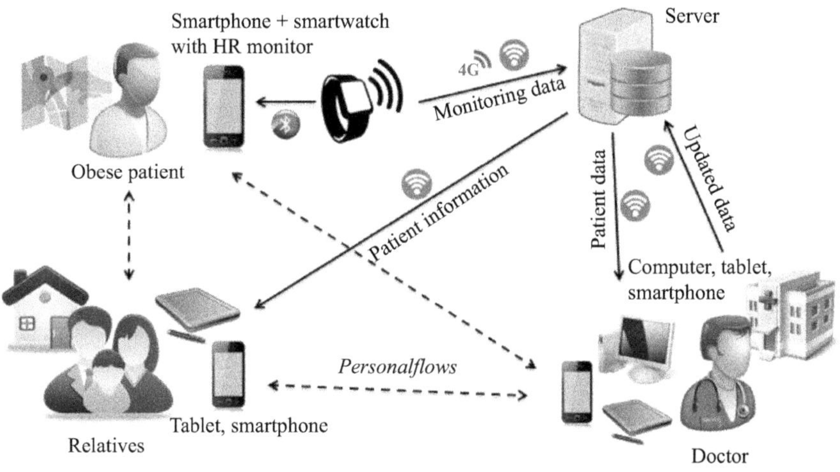

Figure 9.1 Example of mHealth scenario with monitoring objectives

In the example of Figure 9.1, the smartphone of the patient sends data to a server from physical activity gathered by the own smartphone or a smartwatch. These data are analysed by the corresponding algorithms and processes in a server. The doctor can access to the patient information, even data from physical activities in real time by querying the server from a computer, tablet or smartphone. Thus, doctors assess the condition of patient and update information to the server. Besides, relatives and caregivers can know the patient health status by means of their tablets or smartphones. The system also facilitates the self-control of the patient.

Data monitoring is the most important process in monitoring systems, and it is generally characterised by three stages working on obtained data: Data acquisition, Data segmentation and filtering and Data analysis (mainly for continuous signals).

Monitoring process not only works on continuous signals, but also on data from other sources which provide discrete values. Likewise, the processing of data can be carried out by smartphones, computers or servers, depending on the goals and computational requirements.

We have designed and developed mobile systems to monitor several chronic and non-chronic diseases as well as to analyse gait in elderly people. These systems were deployed in simulated and real scenarios to assess different aspects regarding users and the own systems. In the next section, we detail three addressed approaches.

9.4 Vital signs, gait and everyday activities monitoring: experimental applications and study cases

Design of monitoring systems should follow a set of guidelines and common practises to achieve solutions adapted to each particular case. Thus, we have created a scalable framework to develop mobile systems regarding monitoring of a wide group of diseases. Based on this framework, we developed a mobile application to monitor patients with diabetes taking into account glucose level, physical exercise and diet among others. Gait monitoring and analysis is another field in which we have developed several systems to study frailty aspects from gait study. Finally, we also present an analysis tool to monitor Instrumental Activities of Daily Living (IADL) of elderly people who live alone at home as well as several aspects of their caregivers.

9.4.1 Frameworks and mobile systems for chronic and non-chronic diseases

In this section we present a framework based on several layers which is used as a guideline to develop mobile monitoring systems. This include aspects like communication features (between mobile and biometric devices), gathering, processing and storage of data. Generated applications can be useful to create educational material or perform a monitoring of patient with chronic and non-chronic diseases. Besides, we show an approach of a framework-based system to facilitate monitoring tasks, taking into account the clinical profile and a group of health aspects of patients.

9.4.1.1 Description of the system

We have designed a guideline-based solution that allow the development of mobile software architectures through a Mobile Monitoring Framework called MoMo [21]. MoMo offers a solution to facilitate the development and implementation of software architectures and it will facilitate the performance of the activities of people. MoMo implements a solution for devices as mobile phones, PDAs, tablets and any mobile device. The main objective of the framework is to allow the classification, processing and data recovery from generated data of patients to observe fluctuations of normal values of vital signs in accordance with the disease suffered. These values come from mobile devices and biometric measurement devices, which enable the gathering, processing, and storage of data, to be used by other applications, for example, to create educational material, and for prevention and patient monitoring.

The framework defines a complete communication structure (MoMO Layers), a specific ontological classification (MoMo Ontology) [22,23], and a structured pattern definition (MoMo Patterns). Each of these elements allows the integration and creation of different components necessary for the generation of final applications as is shown in Figure 9.2.

With this solution, doctors could examine patients only by consulting their profiles, including the measurements history, generation of statistics (charts) with the patient data [24]. After checking, the application sends the results to the mobile device and the treatment is updated. The treatment can be specific information regarding the disease, generation of diets, intake of medicines and self-control services among others.

We can educate these people about their disease; therefore, an educational component is being developed to allow knowing more about the disease and how to make their daily routines more comfortable. We have a system architecture that allows

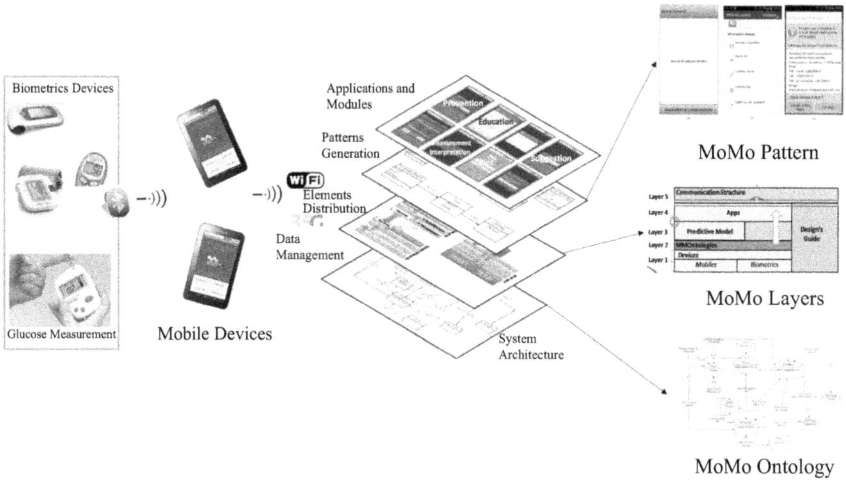

Figure 9.2 Framework structure and main elements used in the development of applications

the patient mobile monitoring through mobile devices. This software architecture is developed through the definition of specific modules; these modules have been developed with a set of patterns that define the user interfaces and the module functionality. We have a layer distribution to send and receive data through mobile devices.

The applications based on the framework are generic, adaptable, remote and mobile. Generic, because they allow the development of applications for multiple diseases following the conceptual design of the developed framework. Adaptable, because they offer services tailored to each type of disease and personalise the user's characteristics, making the interaction more transparent. Remote, because the medical staff can be aware of data obtained by the patient biometric devices through the mobile device in a non-intrusive manner. Mobile, because development is based on the integration of small size, portable and wireless devices. These applications provide greater autonomy for the patient.

Recently, we have proposed a modular framework based on health aspects for monitoring multiple diseases. In this case, the framework determines the interaction with smart devices and smartphones, facilitating patient self-monitoring and clinical treatment. We identified two groups of health aspects: primary and complementary. In the first case, we consider common aspects in most diseases (vital sign, physical activity, clinical record, diet and education); and in the second group are complementary aspects added to improve the disease monitoring (emotions, stress level, environment, etc.) [25]. Figure 9.3 shows the patient monitoring cycle regarding a specific disease, taking into account mobile monitoring scenario presented in Section 9.3.1. The smartphone interacts with smart devices to collect data about vital signs, it is combined with the rest of primary and complementary aspects to support

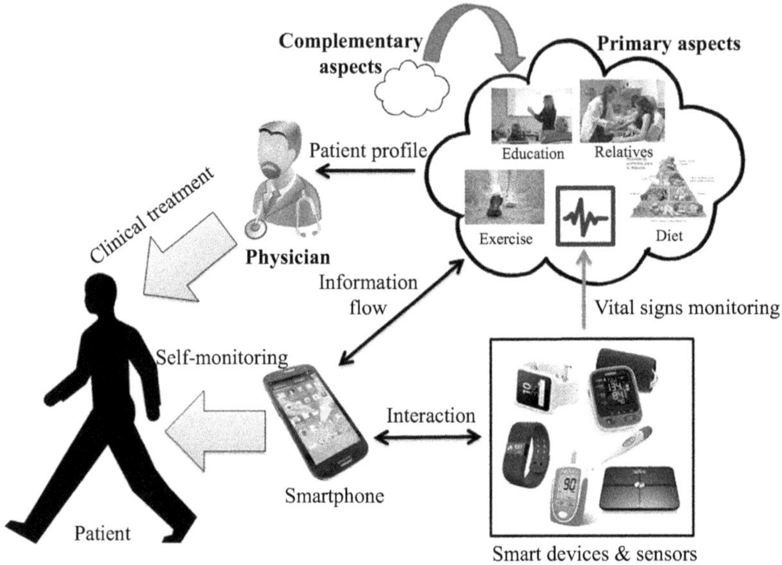

Figure 9.3 Monitoring cycle with interactions and information flows between system elements

self-monitoring. Also, physicians use data from these aspects and the own patient profile to improve the disease's treatment.

These approaches could be the beginning to develop more complex systems related to monitoring behaviour of diseases in which artificial intelligence mechanisms would provide us valuable information about the health condition of patients in real time by using current smart technologies and devices.

9.4.1.2 Evaluation and results

We assessed the impact the system has on patients by developing a mobile application based on the framework. This application allows to store and manage information, and also it provides appropriate recommendations to the patient.

The application was evaluated in 10 patients with diabetes, considering aspects such as the application response time, accuracy of the generated recommendation, assessment of the patient record stored in mobile device, and ease of interaction with the mobile device; all of these characteristics by means of questionnaires delivered to users. We obtained that the response time of the application to the patient is high (90% of answers present a high score and 10% medium score). In the accuracy of the generated recommendation 90% of patients responded with high score and 10% medium, which shows that the application responds according to the patient needs. Another evaluated aspect was the interaction of the patient with the mobile application obtaining high score in 80% of cases.

9.4.2 Long-term gait monitoring as a tool to understand the motor control of gait

Until recently, gait monitoring has been focused on controlled gait trials inside specialised laboratories in physical performance, where it is possible to estimate gait parameters that are both accurate and redundant. These laboratories use highly specialised systems for 3-D motion capture as the Vicon motion capture system (Vicon Motion Systems Ltd., Oxford, UK) or pressure sensorised mats as the GAITRite electronic walkway system (CIR Systems Inc., PA, USA) which provides excellent gait event estimations. Specifically, spatio-temporal gait parameters such as step/stride time and step/stride length are derived from these estimated gait events and summarised through several measures of dispersion in order to characterise person's locomotion at a particular time.

Nonetheless, despite the accuracy achieved by these controlled gait trials to describe the subject's gait condition in a clinical setting, there are a number of constraints that limit their uses and the scope outside the laboratories. In this sense, long-term gait monitoring makes possible to analyse the inherent gait variability over time which is a crucial aspect for diagnosing and monitoring the clinical course of specific disabilities or diseases [26,27]. In such a context, changes in the gait patterns have a potential use as specific predictive markers of frailty syndrome [28,29] and neurodegenerative diseases such as some types of dementia [30,31], among others. From this standpoint, gait evaluations in specialised laboratories are obviously limited over time due to the cost of equipment and the hard deployment of these technologies in a real-life scenario. Consequently, the frequency between gait trials may not be good enough for capturing gait variability with the required time resolution. Furthermore, the subjects who are undergoing the gait trials in the laboratory settings may usually present different gait patterns, feeling conditioned and modifying their walking pace (e.g., increase/decrease the preferred gait velocity, stride time)

Against this background, there is a need for mHealth solutions suitable for characterising gait during daily activities, reducing the stress and anxiety that are present in traditional clinical gait trials. These solutions should get enough gait data to achieve long-term monitoring and to capture the inherent gait variability over time which is useful in understanding the motor control of gait and in providing sound elements to the experts to predict adverse events and diagnose early stages of specific diseases, such as the ones mentioned above.

9.4.2.1 Description of the systems

Developing systems to accurately demarcate gait events such as heel-strike (HS) and toe-off (TO) is a challenging task. Minor changes in the derived gait parameters (e.g., gait velocity, step/stride time) must be properly identified to be able to capture gait variability. In terms of sensor deployment strategies, gait events can be detected through deploying sensors in the environment and making them ambient and stationary. This is the case for most of the vision systems for gait monitoring [32]. Other approaches are based on wearable devices which can be divided according to the anatomical reference used to set the sensors, since this determines the way gait events are obtained. The simplest scheme uses a single inertial unit to get trunk acceleration, estimating gait events from these measurements through the use of a wide set of techniques [33]. A dedicated inertial sensor is usually placed between L1–L3 vertebrae to measure trunk acceleration and angular velocity during the gait. In other cases, instead of a dedicated sensor, the inertial measurement unit integrated in a mobile phone is used. However, to demarcate the exact timestamp of each gait event the phone must also be fixed to the lumbar zone using a customised belt and therefore the resulting ambulatory system is far from being non-intrusive [34].

Whether adopting a stationary deployment strategy with environment sensors or an ambulatory and nomadic approach through wearables and built-in mobile phone sensors, gait monitoring services drawn as mHealth systems receive the benefits of using mobile phones, either as part of the sensorisation, data processing or through their use as end-devices where relevant information is communicated to patients, relatives and clinicians.

The rest of this section describes two systems for long-term gait monitoring in household and community contexts in which we are currently working on. The first one is a stationary approach using a structured light sensor to capture gait trajectories passively from the camera scene, identifying straight paths and monitoring gait activity inside them. The second one is a proposal for a wearable inertial sensor infrastructure using a MQTT[1] topology, commonly utilised in IoT.[2] This will allow us to monitor the gait of several elders in a residential environment throughout the day.

Passive vision-based system for gait monitoring

This is a computer vision system based on the utilisation of a low-cost structured light sensor, particularly a Kinect 1 device (Microsoft Corporation, WA, USA), to externally estimate HS events. This is done by tracking 3D point-clouds relative to human bodies within the scene and then applying a pass-through filter to cut off points from each human's point-cloud that correspond to the lower limbs (see Figure 9.4(a)). The centroid locations from the lower limb point-clouds are used to estimate the gait trajectories over time.

As gait trajectories could include turns or abrupt changes of direction, a two-stage straightness analysis is also performed to extract straight paths. Like most of the clinical gait trials, only linear/straight paths are considered because turns or abrupt changes in the trajectory distort the measurements obtained during the gait assessment. In Figure 9.4(a), a single straight path (solid line) has been identified, as the subject is transversely crossing the scene in only one direction.

After identifying the straight paths within a gait trajectory, the lower limb point-clouds enclosed by each of these paths are projected onto the floor plane (drawing up something similar to a set of "footfalls", see Figure 9.4(b)). Each projection is then normalised and aligned to the concerned path line. Finally, the Pearson correlation coefficient is computed for each of the normalised projections belonging to

[1]MQTT or Message Queuing Telemetry Transport is a connectivity protocol designed as an extremely lightweight publish/subscribe messaging transport.
[2]Internet of Things.

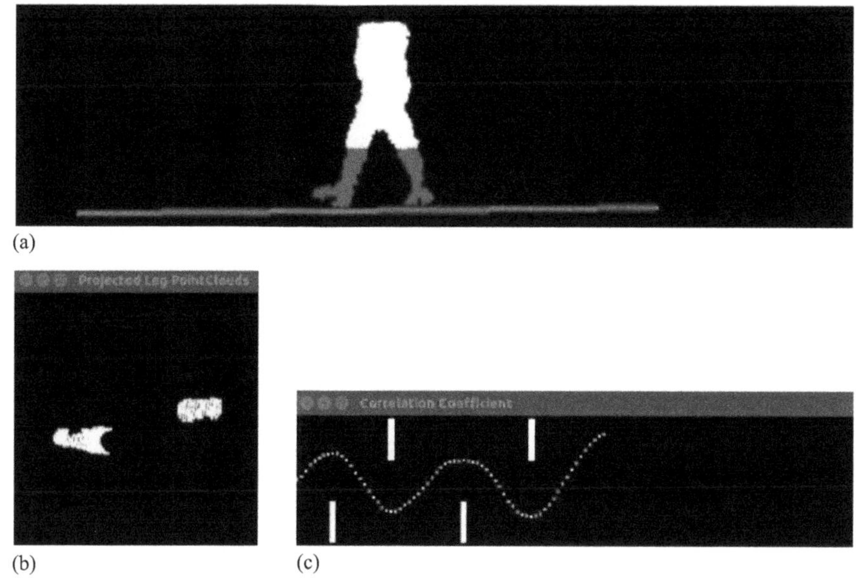

Figure 9.4 *Passive vision-based system for gait monitoring. (a) 3D view displaying a human point-cloud (light hue), the segmented lower limb point-cloud (dark hue) and the identified straight path (solid line). (b) Normalised and aligned lower limb projection (footfalls). (c) Filtered Pearson's correlation coefficient time series. Local maxima correspond to left heel strikes and local minima to right heel strikes*

the same straight path, composing together a correlation time series. After applying a filter combining Gaussian kernels of different size, HS events are located at the maximum and minimum peaks of the smoothed correlation time series. Step and stride times are directly computed from the HS demarcations. Moreover, using the duration and length of each straight path, gait velocity and cadence estimations are also provided. In Figure 9.4(c), one part of the filtered Pearson's correlation time series is displayed, from the beginning of the gait trial until the time prior to a left HS (local maximum).

The main advantage of using this kind of approach based on a structured light sensor combined with point-cloud processing is the improvement achieved in terms of robustness to the sensor's location. Flexibility when placing the vision sensor inside the living environment is definitely a key point in order to provide long-term in-home gait monitoring, enabling the acquisition of gait measurements passively in the course of the day. Therefore, the proposed vision-based solution should return similar performance in gait parameter estimations under different scenarios if, for example, the sensor is located next to the room's roof or at half the height of the wall, as long as the potential walking area is captured without occlusions.

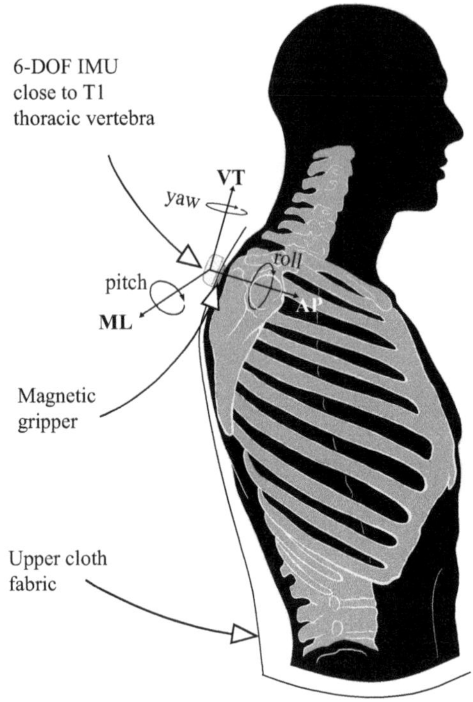

Figure 9.5 IMU attached using the magnetic grip system. The vertical (VT), antero-posterior (AP), medio-lateral (ML) axes and the Euler angles (yaw/pitch/roll) are displayed

The system has been described in detail in [35] and compared with regard to a reference clinical instrument (GAITRite) under controlled trials to validate the feasibility of estimating temporal gait parameters with it. More details are provided in the Results section.

Proposal of an inertial sensor infrastructure for long-term gait monitoring and stride-to-stride fluctuation analysis in a residential environment

This approach intends to monitor the gait of several elders in a residential environment throughout the day and without any human intervention during gait data acquisition. Unlike the previous system, an ambulatory approach is proposed here using an infrastructure composed of wearable devices which are attached to the upper cloth of each elderly subject by means of a magnetic gripper, close to the T1 thoracic vertebra as shown in the diagram in Figure 9.5.

Each wearable device is equipped with a small 802.11 wireless transmitter ESP-826612E (Espressif Systems Inc., Shanghai, China), which integrates a 32-bit RISC Tensilica Xtensa LX106 micro-controller that enables I^2C communication[3] with a

[3]Inter-Integrated Circuit data serial bus.

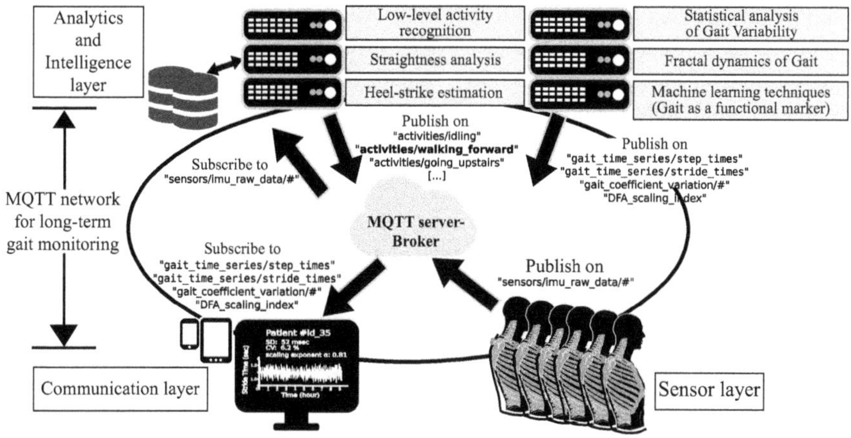

Figure 9.6 Overview of the MQTT network infrastructure

single InvenSense MPU-6050 6-DOF IMU[4] (InvenSense Inc., CA, USA). This setup allows us to acquire trunk accelerations and trunk orientations during walking for each of the elders at 100 Hz uniform sample rate and transmit them to a dedicated server (broker) using the MQTT messaging protocol, commonly implemented in IoT networks for managing sensor data transmissions. An overview of this approach is shown in Figure 9.6.

A special client is subscribed to the "`sensors/imu_raw_data/#`" topic, receiving raw data from trunk accelerations and orientations in order to provide reasoning capabilities to discriminate walking forward from other low-level activities, such as idling, going upstairs, going downstairs, rotating on the subject's axis and running. A Gaussian Naive Bayes (GNB) classifier similar to the one proposed in [36] enables low-level activity clustering. In this case, the feature vector is composed of time domain and spectral features derived from trunk accelerations and orientations (e.g., sum of acceleration magnitude below 25 percentile, peak frequency in vertical acceleration below 5 Hz, number of peaks in spectrum below 5 Hz)

From those periods of activity identified as "walking forward periods", a straightness analysis procedure, considering the changes in yaw rotation, is conducted to identify turns or changes of direction which are required to properly segment the straight paths inside the gait trajectory. Raw data produced while walking through each of these segmented straight paths feed a modified version of the algorithm presented in [34], used to estimated HS events from trunk acceleration signals through scale-space filtering. Gait parameter time series derived from HS events, such as step/stride time series are published on the "`gait_time_series/#`" topic. Different kinds of clients, such as mobile phones or computers may subscribe to this topic

[4]Six-Degrees of Freedom Inertial Measurement Unit (three-axis accelerometer and three-axis gyroscope).

to communicate this information to patients, relatives and clinicians. Furthermore, reasoning capabilities at this data processing level can help to characterise person's locomotion over time, either based on a statistical analysis of dispersion or by using more novel approaches such as fractal dynamics to analyse long-range correlations in stride interval fluctuations [37].

9.4.2.2 Evaluation and results

Passive vision-based system for gait monitoring

An experimental protocol has been designed and conducted to compare the gait parameters[5] estimated through the vision-based system with regard to a GAITRite walkway. Eight female and two male subjects, with ages from 18 to 80 years and no evidence of gait disorder or known limitation have participated in the experiment. The subjects have been divided into two groups of ages, five elders (age: 68.2 ± 6 years) and five young subjects (age: 24.4 ± 5.3 years).

For validating purposes, the Kinect device was 240 cm separated from the GAITRite capturing a sagittal view of the subjects during the gait trials. Two height configurations were tested (at 65 cm from the floor and at 240 cm). For each of the height configurations, all the subjects walked on the GAITRite five times; the first and the last were gait trials with no data collected. Therefore, six gait trials were recorded for each participant. Absolute and relative errors with respect to the GAITRite were computed, being the step time for the older group the gait parameter with more relative error (around $4\% \pm 3.5$), dealing with values of absolute error below 50 ms for the two height configurations.

The comparison under controlled conditions performed in [35] is a required stage to validate the feasibility of estimating temporal gait parameters with this vision-based approach, previous to its deployment in Ambient Assisted Living environments and its evaluation to provide long-term in-home gait monitoring, in which we are currently working on.

Inertial sensor infrastructure for long-term gait monitoring and stride-to-stride fluctuation analysis in a residential environment

The proposal presented here is under development to this day. A reduced number of working prototypes of the wearable device have been built and integrated in a small MQTT network for testing purposes. The *low-level activity recognition*, the *straightness analysis* and the *heel-strike estimation* modules (see Figure 9.6) have been implemented as part of the *Analytics and Intelligence layer*. Preliminary results from the evaluation of these modules in a residential environment will be published in the next months.

9.4.3 Analysis tools for monitoring

The scope of monitoring term goes beyond monitoring physical activities or diseases. There are other activities that can be monitored. In this sense, we developed a software system, based on software modules, in the context of the Personal IADL Assistant

[5] Step and stride time.

(PIA) project[6] to monitor a subset of IADL of elderly people who live alone at home [38]. Thus, healthcare researchers and caregivers had access to valuable information about the activities carried out by their elders. Also, the system gathered information about the own caregivers to measure their burden and stress level by means of different surveys.

9.4.3.1 Description of the system

The system is presented as an analysis tool based on a theoretical model and a methodology (presented in [38]) to develop software tools for analysing everyday activities of users and several aspects of caregivers. The information for the analysis come from two different sources: (a) from interaction between elder and environmental elements and (b) from the direct application of questionnaires to the caregiver. The system collects information from these sources and provides a support to researchers in the analysis of IADL, carer stress and quality of life (QoL) levels.

The software communicates with other tools and applications to acquire relevant information from users. For example, external applications provide information about the interactions between users and elements of the environment. In a specific context, users generate implicit and explicit information when they interact with other elements; these elements can be physical objects (e.g. washing machine) or software applications. Thus, when an user interacts with an element of the environment, certain valuable information can be generated and saved. These data are considered system inputs used for the later analysis.

Figure 9.7 shows an example of collecting information from the interaction between an elder and a tablet device. In this case, a video clip explaining how the medication should be taken is displayed on the tablet when the elder touches the specific environmental object (e.g. in this case a Near Field Communication[7] tag attached to the medication box). While playing the video, the user could press on the home button and this information is sent to the analysis tool. Then, caregivers and researchers will be able to visualise that information for their purposes.

Furthermore, the analysis tool provides a software module to generate questionnaires and collect the results. This part of the system contributes to collect factual data in order to assess several aspects regarding IADL performance, carer stress and QoL of elders and caregivers. We developed a questionnaires-based engine to facilitate the management of tests and gathering of their results. Thus, schema of the questionnaires, interpretation and recommendations based on scores were saved into the analysis system. These tests are interactive and dynamic, where the answers given during its completion modify the followed path and the final results. Depending on the path, the results are different and the user receives different recommendations.

9.4.3.2 Evaluation and results

The analysis tool was deployed in an elderly context for supporting caregivers of elderly people to promote the performance of IADL and improve the QoL of elders

[6] http://pia-project.org
[7] http://www.nearfieldcommunication.org/

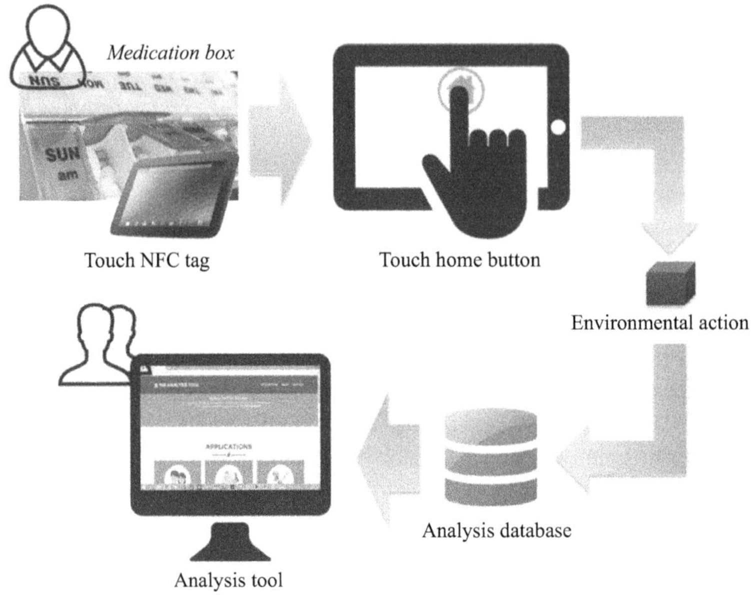

Figure 9.7 Example of IADL information gathering when the user presses on a mobile app button

and carers, as well as to reduce the stress level on caregivers. In the environment, we identified three types of users: elders, caregivers and therapists. The software modules for caregivers and therapists were evaluated on ten users by means of two evaluation protocols. Both protocols consist of using the corresponding module, trying all its features and completing an agreement-based survey to collect feedback from the software use. The aspects evaluated were the following: Comprehension of the functionalities, Intuitiveness and consistency of interface elements, Design of visual components, Comprehension and relevance of the analysis, Usefulness level and ease of interpretation of the results.

According to the assessment results, 90% of users think that the user interface of the software modules is clear and simple. Eighty-five per cent of users determine the suitability of the information provided. Caregivers said that the questionnaires to be completed were easy to answer and still clear and easy to navigate due to their responsive approach. However, 10% of caregivers thought that some resulting recommendations were unclear. Obviously, it depended on the therapist who created the questionnaire with the tool.

On the other hand, functionalities regarding monitoring of elder interactions proved to be useful for 95% of caregivers. Most caregivers assessed as positive in the feedback provided by the software tool to promote the improvement of QoL aspects. Also, statistical information showed was very relevant for therapists.

We have seen how reliability and effectiveness of some parts of the system (those showing questionnaires) depend on therapists or people who make the questionnaires to be completed by caregivers. This tool provided the fundamentals to enable a deeper analysis and an appropriate clinical treatment.

9.5 Conclusions

In this chapter, we have shown an overview about the current state of mobile monitoring in assisted environments. From the Ambient Intelligent paradigm, it is possible to provide smart services in healthcare scenarios. With the growth of mobile technologies appears the concept of mHealth. Thus, mHealth refers to the use and deployment of these services and systems by using mobile devices and wireless networks in health environments.

One of the most important approaches in mHealth domain corresponds to mobile monitoring. Currently, monitoring of health parameters is widely used in our society due to commercial devices such as smartphones, bracelets and smartwatches. Thus, development of systems in this research area provides users mechanisms to improve diseases monitoring providing clinical benefits.

We have developed three different monitoring systems focused on monitoring of chronic and non-chronic diseases, gait monitoring and analysis of IADL tasks.

In the first case, we presented a framework that allows the generation of mobile applications for monitoring patient diseases. We can adapt the applications to patient requirements providing different modules for diet, recommendations, education and alerts depending on the last measures obtained through the communication between biometric devices and mobiles devices. This module sends the measurement to predictive inference engine for the interpretation and adaptation of the new modules. The evaluation related to the time of response, suggestions generated and the application interaction presented a high score for the evaluated patients.

For the long-term gait monitoring, we have presented two approaches, the first one consists of a passive vision-based system using a structured light sensor which can be placed stationary anywhere in the house, as long as potential walking areas are captured without occlusions; the second one is a proposal of a MQTT network infrastructure composed of inertial-based devices to be placed on the thoracic zone of elderly people. Both approaches can acquire temporal gait parameters such as step/stride times throughout the day and without any human intervention. Gait variability analysis are conducted in the respective intelligence layers providing relevant information about the motor control of gait that enables the use of long-term gait monitoring as a predictive marker of adverse events or to diagnose early stages of specific diseases. In both cases, mobile phones may be used as end-point communication devices with patients, relatives and clinicians.

Finally we described an analysis tool with different software modules to be integrated in assistive systems. The aim of this software tool was to collect relevant information about elderly people who live alone at home and their caregivers. This was achieved through several components that gathered factual information from environmental interactions between elders and different appliances, and also from questionnaires completed by caregivers to measure stress and QoL levels.

According to these systems and the works from the literature, the idea of involving physicians, caregivers and patients in a multi-monitoring smart context is getting closer.

Acknowledgements

This work has been supported by the coordinated project *FRASE*, granted by the Spanish Ministerio de Ciencia e Innovación, and by the UBIHEALTH project under the International Research Staff Exchange Schema program (MC-IRSES 316337). This work has also been funded by Castilla-La Mancha University under the *Plan Propio de Investigación* program and supported by Fundación Mapfre.

References

[1] P. Filipe and N. Mamede, A task repository for ambient intelligence, *Natural Language Processing and Information Systems*. Germany, Springer, 2006, vol. 3999, pp. 70–81. doi: 10.1007/11765448_7, 2006.
[2] M. Weiser, "Some computers science issues in ubiquitous computing," *Commun. ACM*, vol. 36, pp. 75–84, 1993.
[3] M. Coen, "Design principles for intelligent environments," in *AAAI Spring Symposium on Intelligent Environments*, USA, California, pp. 547–554, 1998.
[4] A. Nijholt, T. Rist, and Tuijnenbreijer, "Lost in ambient intelligence?" in *CHI'04 Extended Abstracts on Human Factors in Computing Systems*, 2004, pp. 1725–1726.
[5] E. Aarts, R. Harwig, and M. Schuurmans, Ambient intelligence, *The Invisible Future: The Seamless Integration of Technology into Everyday Life*. USA, McGraw Hill, 2002, ch. Ambient Intelligence, pp. 235–250.
[6] A. Talukder and R. Yavagal, *Mobile Computing: Technology, Applications, and Service Creation*, USA, McGraw-Hill, 2007.
[7] U. Varshney, "Pervasive healthcare," *IEEE Comput.*, vol. 36, no. 12, pp. 138–140, 2003.
[8] WHO, "mhealth. new horizons for health through mobile technologies," World Health Organization (WHO), Tech. Rep., 2011.
[9] R. Istepanian and J. Lacal, "Emerging mobile communication technologies for health: some imperative notes on m-health," *Eng. Med. Biol. Soc., 2003*, 2003,
[10] N. Lane, E. Miluzo, H. Lu, and D. Peebles, "A survey of mobile phone sensing," *Commun. Mag.*, USA, IEEE, vol. 48, no. 9, pp. 140–150, 2010.
[11] M. Mun, S. Reddy, S. K. N. Yau, *et al.*, "Peir, the personal environmental impact report, as a platform for participatory sensing systems research," in *Proceedings of International Conference on Mobile Systems, Applications, and Services*, 2009, pp. 55–68.

[12] R. Istepanian, C. Pattichis, and S. Laxminarayan, Ubiquitous M-Health systems and the convergence towards 4G mobile technologies. *M-Health. Emerging Mobile Health Systems*. Germany, Springer, 2006, pp. 3–14.
[13] S. Laxminarayan and I. R., "Unwired e-med: the next generation of wireless and internet telemedicine systems," *IEEE Trans. Inf. Technol. Biomed.*, vol. 4, no. 3, pp. 189–193, 2000.
[14] E. Jovanov, A. Lords, D. Raskovic, P. Cox, R. Adhami, and F. Andrasik, "Stress monitoring using a distributed wireless intelligent sensor system," *IEEE Eng. Med. Biol. Mag.*, vol. 22, no. 3, pp. 49–55, 2003.
[15] C. Pattichis, E. Kyriacou, S. Voskarides, M. Pattichis, R. Istepanian, and C. Schizas, "Wireless telemedicine systems: an overview," *IEEE Antenn. Propag.*, vol. 44, no. 2, pp. 143–153, 2002.
[16] S. Tachakra, X. Wang, R. Istepanian, and Y. Song, "Mobile e-health: the unwired evolution of telemedicine," *Telemed. J. e-Health*, vol. 9, no. 3, pp. 247–257, 2003.
[17] J. Lee, "Smart health: concepts and status of ubiquitous health with smartphone," in *International Conference on ICT Convergence (ICTC) Proceedings*, Seoul, Corea., USA, IEEE, 2011.
[18] A. Kwan, "Using mobile technologies for heatlhier aging," mHealth Alliance. United Nations Foundation, 2012.
[19] A. Willis, "The ecosystem: an evolving concept viewed historically," *Funct. Ecol.*, vol. 11, no. 2, pp. 268–271, 1997.
[20] D. Boecker, B. Mikoleit, and D. Scheffer, "mHealth and population management," *mHealth. Multidisciplinary Verticals*. USA, CRC, 2015, pp. 157–180.
[21] V. Villarreal, R. Hervas, F. Fontecha, and J. Bravo, "Mobile monitoring framework to design parameterized and personalized m-health applications according to the patient's diseases," *J. Med. Syst.*, vol. 39, no. 132, pp. 1–6, 2015.
[22] V. Villarreal, R. Hervas, A. Diez, and J. Bravo, "Applying ontologies in the development of patient mobile monitoring framework," in *Second International Conference on e-Health and Bioengineering (EHB)*, Constanta (Romania). USA, IEEE, 2009.
[23] M. Fernandez-Lopez, "Overview of methodology for building ontologies," in *Workshop on Ontologies and Problem-Solving Methods: Lessons Learned and Future Trends (IJCAI)*, Stockholm, Sweeden, 1999.
[24] V. Villarreal, J. Laguna, S. Lopez, *et al.*, "A proposal for mobile diabetes self-control: towards a patient monitoring framework," in *Distributed Computing, Artificial Intelligence, Bioinformatics, Soft Computing and Ambient Assisted Living (IWANN)*, vol. 5518. Germany, Springer, 2009, pp. 870–877.
[25] J. Fontecha, R. Hervas, and J. Bravo, "A sensorized and health aspect-based framework to improve the continuous monitoring on diseases using smartphones and smart devices," in *Ambient Intelligence for Health (First International Conference AmIHealth)*, J. Bravo, R. Hervas, and V. Villarreal, Eds., vol. 9456. Germany, Springer, 2015, pp. 68–73.

[26] J. Brach, S. Perera, S. Studenski, and A. Newman, "The reliability and validity of measures of gait variability in community-dwelling older adults," *Arch. Phys. Med. Rehabil.*, vol. 89, no. 12, pp. 2293–2296, 2008.

[27] J. Hausdorff, "Gait variability: methods, modeling and meaning," *J. NeuroEng. Rehabil.*, vol. 2, no. 19, 2005.

[28] J. Fontecha, F. Navarro, R. Hervas, and J. Bravo, "Elderly frailty detection by using accelerometer-enabled smartphones and clinical information records," *J. Pers. Ubiquit. Comput.*, vol. 17, no. 6, pp. 1073–1083, 2013.

[29] M. Montero-Odasso, S. Muir, M. Hall, *et al.*, "Gait variability is associated with frailty in community-dwelling older adults," *J. Gerontol. A. Biol. Sci. Med. Sci.*, vol. 66, no. 5, pp. 568–576., 2011.

[30] J. Verghese, R. Lipton, and C. Hall, "Abnormality of gait as a predictor of non-Alzheimer's dementia," *N. Engl. J. Med.*, vol. 347, no. 22, pp. 1761–1768, 2002.

[31] L. Waite, D. Grayson, O. Piguet, H. Creasey, H. Bennett, and G. Broe, "Gait slowing as a predictor of incident dementia: 6-year longitudinal data from the Sydney older persons study," *J. Neurol. Sci.*, vol. 229–230, pp. 89–93, 2005.

[32] A. Muro-de-la Herran, B. Garcia-Zapirain, and A. Mendez-Zorrilla, "Gait analysis methods: an overview of wearable and non-wearable systems, highlighting clinical applications," *Sensors*, vol. 14, no. 2, pp. 3362–3394, 2014.

[33] D. Trojaniello, A. Ravaschio, J. Hausdorff, and A. Cereatti, "Comparative assessment of different methods for the estimation of gait temporal parameters using a single inertial sensor: application to elderly, post-stroke, Parkinson's disease and Huntington's disease subjects," *Gait & Posture*, vol. 42, no. 3, pp. 310–316, 2015.

[34] I. González, J. Fontecha, R. Hervás, and J. Bravo, "Estimation of temporal gait events from a single accelerometer through scale-space filtering," *J. Med. Syst.*, vol. 40, no. 251, 2016.

[35] I. González, I. López-Nava, J. Fontecha, A. Muñoz-Meléndez, A. Pérez-Sanpablo, and I. Quiñones-Urióstegui, "Comparison between passive vision-based system and a wearable inertial-based system for estimating temporal gait parameters related to the GAITRite electronic walkway." *J. Biomed. Inf.*, vol. 62, no. C, pp. 210–223, 2016.

[36] I. González, J. Fontecha, R. Hervás, and J. Bravo, "An ambulatory system for gait monitoring based on wireless sensorized insoles," *Sensors*, vol. 15, no. 7, pp. 16 589–16 613, 2015.

[37] J. Hausdorff, "Gait dynamics, fractals and falls: finding meaning in the stride-to-stride fluctuations of human walking," *Hum. Move. Sci.*, vol. 26, no. 4, pp. 555–589, 2007.

[38] J. Fontecha, R. Hervas, P. Mondejar, I. González, and J. Bravo, "Towards context-aware and user-centered analysis in assistive environments," *J. Med. Syst.*, vol. 39, no. 120, 2015.

Chapter 10

Smartphone-based blood pressure monitoring for falls risk assessment: techniques and technologies

Hamid GholamHosseini, Mirza Mansoor Baig, Andries Meintjes, Farhaan Mirza, and Maria Lindén

Abstract

Smart patient monitoring systems have rapidly evolved during the past two decades and have the potential to improve current patient care and medical staff workflow. With advanced sensors, sophisticated hardware and fast-growing wireless communication technologies, there are enormous opportunities for ubiquitous solutions in all areas of healthcare, especially patient monitoring.

Current methods of non-invasive blood pressure measurement are based on inflation and deflation of a cuff with some effects on arteries where blood pressure is being measured. This approach is non-continuous, time delayed, and might cause patient discomfort. We aim to monitor and measure cuff-less and continuous blood pressure using a smartphone. Cuff-less approach enables continuous blood pressure monitoring capabilities and is particularly attractive as blood pressure is one of the most important factors to assess risk of falls in older adults.

A smartphone application was developed to collect PhotoPlethysmoGram (PPG) waveform and electrocardiogram (ECG) in order to calculate pulse transit time (PTT). The user's systolic blood pressure is calculated using the PPT and precise optimisation model. The proposed application can be integrated with our developed falls risk assessment algorithm for inpatient older adults. This study proposes a novel approach of continuous blood pressure monitoring using cuff-less method that can be employed for prevention of inpatient falls using smartphone.

Keywords

Smartphone health application, Falls risk assessment, mHealth monitoring, Cuff-less blood pressure monitoring, Continuous blood pressure monitoring

10.1 Introduction

Tablets and smartphones as ubiquitous devices are now becoming important part of human life and healthcare-related services [1]. Smartphones provide high computing power of a personal computer as well as wireless and cellular connectivity of a mobile phone with compact size, fast processing, and several in-built sensors and features that are useful for clinical settings. They can be employed by health professionals for administration, billing, health information, appointments, laboratory results and clinical quality matrix [1–3].

With the advent of mobile communications using smartphones, their high computing power has been the main driver of research and development of ubiquitous applications (apps). It offers tremendous potential to create efficient smartphone-based solutions [4] to deliver healthcare anytime and anywhere, surpassing geographical, temporal, and even organisational barriers. Smartphone-based healthcare applications and their corresponding mobility functionalities tend to have a strong impact on typical healthcare monitoring, decision support, and alerting systems [4].

The ultimate success of mobile healthcare systems in hospital care settings is still debatable [5,6]. There are very limited studies on successful implementation and/or clinically trailed system in wider hospital care settings. Monitoring devices that previously could only be found in hospital wards and doctors' offices are now available in more compact and affordable packages [7]. The development of these devices is being driven partly by the greater need for affordable, reliable, and convenient methods of personal health monitoring due to both the aging population in much of the developed world as well as the increasing burden of chronic disease [8].

Blood pressure is often monitored by medical professionals along with body temperature, pulse rate and respiration rate as a main vital sign that is useful in detecting or predicting medical problems. Majority of the blood pressure monitors operate using an inflatable cuff and oscillatory method to calculate a patient's blood pressure intermittently. This method has several drawbacks, such as the cuff inflating and deflating is cumbersome and irritating, and blood pressure measurements are limited to a certain period or time. *Continuous* blood pressure monitoring has diagnostic advantages over periodic measurements, since blood pressure may change abruptly during conditions such as falls or exercise. These varying measurements often have more diagnostic value than a typical time-based instantaneous blood pressure readings. Currently, continuous methods of blood pressure monitoring make use of invasive catheters with pressure sensors attached inserted directly into an artery where the pressure is measured [9].

Recent studies indicate an inverse correlation between the time taken by a pulse wave produced by the heart to reach peripheral capillaries (pulse transit times) and blood pressure. Although the results of these studies vary in quality, the overall consensus is that pulse transit time (PTT) can be used as an indicator of arterial blood pressure [9,10].

The PTT can be estimated by finding the time difference between the R wave of an electrocardiogram (ECG) and the corresponding peak of a PhotoPlethysmoGram (PPG) waveform provided by a pulse oximeter. This time is then related to pulse wave velocity by taking into account the approximate distance travelled by the pulse wave. For this research, the pre-ejection period was disregarded, and the peak of the PPG waveform was used in the calculation of the PTT. This could influence the quality of the results, especially in cases where the pre-ejection period is extended because of medication or disease [2,3,11,12].

Dropping blood pressure is one of the main contributing factors to the risk of falls in hospitalised patients. We have included the changes of blood pressure and other vital signs into a multifactorial falls risk assessment model where motion activity and patient health record are also considered to capture patient's activities and changes in health conditions.

10.2 Mobile healthcare applications

Smartphones are emerging as evidence-based tools designed to help clinical workflow, clinician decision making and patient participation in making specific and deliberate choices among healthcare options [13]. The International Patient Decision Aids Standards (IPDAS) identifies key components and standards of a high-quality patient decision aid [14]. Most of mobile applications offer four basic advantages: (1) data sharing; (2) data organisation (alerts and history); (3) decision support/interpretation; (4) user knowledge and support. Those advantages of smartphone apps lead to the integration of electronic medical record (EMR) and/or electronic patient record (EPR) with various mobile devices [15].

10.2.1 Smartphone applications in the secondary care

Manual paper or hardcopy based healthcare assessments can be automated with easy to use Graphical User Interface (GUI) via smartphone applications. This approach of creating a digital and mobile technology platform to capture essential assessment data is common, which contributes to consistency and accuracy in clinical documentation. For example, a smartphone based application for wound care [16] was developed to replicate the paper-based Pressure Ulcer Scale for Healing (PUSH tool) [17], Braden Scale [18] and the Bates-Jensen tool [19]. This system automated the existing tools and allowed clinicians to create, view, access, delete and re-assess patient records. Critical design consideration is applied to the smartphone application including: simplicity of GUI; minimising visual elements on any given screen to reduce clutter; using colour cues to focus information and converging on critical information. It is also reported that the number of steps to complete a common task related to wound care is significantly reduced using mHealth tools. The application was developed for a Nexus 4 smartphone and Nexus 7 tablet and tested with eight nurses, age range 31–60 years. There was a very strong perceived correlation between the paper-based forms and the wound care app in terms of content and data entry expectations, with scores of 4.60/5.00 for the Braden Scale and 4.57/5.00 for the PUSH tool [16]. However, there is privacy and security concerns regarding effective use and governance of clinical data stored by the entities, departments, or organisations by the nationalised data-sharing schemes [20].

However, often such applications act as isolated systems for healthcare professionals to be used for specific purposes. This creates the issue of usability and integration with other healthcare systems.

10.2.2 Application of tablets and smartphones in monitoring of daily activities of hospitalised patients

A randomised controlled trial was conducted to compare the efficacy of a computerised physical activity program [21], where older adult patients were given a tablet computer for the initial two months to enter their daily activity data using a simple GUI. Two-hundred and sixty-three older adults were recruited from three outpatient clinics at Boston Medical Centre with average age of 65 years. It was reported that there was a higher rate of pedometer data capture in the control group after 12 months of trial (52.5% vs 39.6%). It was also notable that the tablet decline rate of the users was at an average of 35.8 ± 19.7 times during the 60-day in-home intervention phase, and after the first week (from an average of 4.7 to 4.0 sessions/week) and then gradually declining (to 3.3 sessions/week). Most of mHealth applications are designed without clinician or end user consultations. Therefore, they are prone to issues such as application usage, especially for older adults who may have difficulty understanding the application and/or handling the tablet application [22] – which potentially reducing the global adoption of mobile applications [23,24].

10.3 Design and methodology of the smart monitoring application

10.3.1 Medical device and wireless connectivity

Wireless medical devices used in this research have the capability of collecting blood pressure (BP), acceleration, ECG and pulse wave synchronously from multiple patients. Figure 10.1 shows the architectural diagram of a smartphone application which collects real-time data from the available wireless medical devices and transfers either the alerts or the raw data to other devices. Depending upon the clinician's

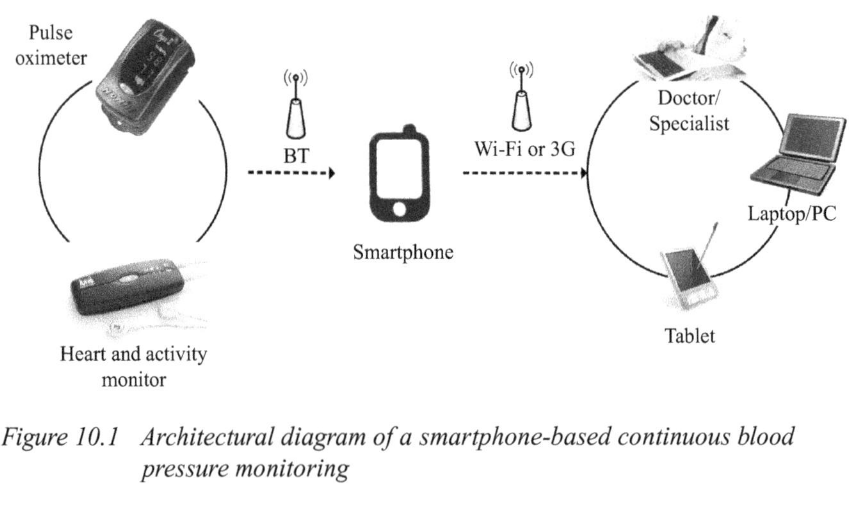

Figure 10.1 Architectural diagram of a smartphone-based continuous blood pressure monitoring

requirement and configuration, the alerts and raw data can be restricted for a mobile devices, laptops, or smartphones. The Alive Heart and Activity Monitor and the Nonin Pulse Oximeter were used to acquire ECG and PPG signals. The Alive Heart and Activity Monitor includes a 2-lead ECG and accelerometer in a lightweight and portable package. This device is powered using a rechargeable battery and includes support for Bluetooth version 2.1 using Serial Port Profile (SPP). The ECG has a sampling rate of 300 Hz with an 8-bit resolution [25]. The Nonin Pulse Oximeter has a sampling rate of 75 Hz and includes support for Bluetooth transmission. The data format for this device was set up so that the plethysmograph information, peripheral perfusion percentage, and the heart rate of the person is continuously streamed from the device.

10.3.2 Continuous blood pressure monitoring applications

The Alive Bluetooth Heart and Activity Monitor with single channel ECG and an in-built three axes accelerometer was used to collect ECG signals. This device can be connected to other mobile devices over the standard Bluetooth interface with a range of up to 100 m for real-time transmission of ECG and accelerometer data. It can also save data on internal device storage (1 GB SD card) for offline analysis.

The incoming data samples from both the devices are acquired, processed by the QRS and peak detection algorithms and then passed on to the activity logger which displays the processed data in a meaningful way. The number of samples received from each device is stored under the user's historic trend and timeline of the significant health deteriorations. The Nonin pulse oximeter has a delay (nominally five seconds) after the connection is established via Bluetooth and before the data transmission starts. The start of the ECG data transmission is set as a time line and considered to be time zero. The data samples are converted to their expected real-time value based on the sampling rate of the devices. The pulse oximeter samples are shifted forward by 5 s to match for the transmission time delay.

When a QRS complex is detected, its time index is stored in an array. When the peak detection algorithm detects a peak in the PPG waveform the peak time is compared with the stored time of related QRS in the array. The smallest positive difference between the PPG peak time and one of the QRS complexes is considered as the PTT for that beat as shown in (10.1).

$$\mathrm{PTT} = \mathrm{PPG\ peak\ time} - \mathrm{QRS\ complex\ time\ [ms]} \tag{10.1}$$

This PTT is then used to calculate the pulse wave velocity (PWV) of the user, which is directly related to the user's blood pressure. The PTT of the person can be related to the PWV using (10.2).

$$\mathrm{PWV} = 0.5 \cdot \mathrm{Height}/\mathrm{PTT\ [cm/ms]} \tag{10.2}$$

where a finger pulse oximeter is being used and the height of the person is in centimetres and the PTT in milliseconds.

10.3.3 System calibration and optimization

In order to estimate absolute values of systolic blood pressure the system is calibrated using an external blood pressure monitor while PTT is being measured in real-time. The critical issue of time delay is achieved by starting the PTT measurements first and then initiating the calibration procedure on the Alive Heart and Activity Monitor.

When the blood pressure measurement is completed the user is required to press the event button and enters the systolic blood pressure measured by the external blood pressure monitor. This calibration process is heavily reliant on the signals from the pulse oximeter and the heart monitor being clear and noise free, thus it is critical that the ECG probes be firmly connected to the patient and the pulse oximeter be kept completely still during this process. This procedure allows the system to calculate a calibration coefficient as shown in (10.3).

$$\text{Calibration Coefficient (CC)} = BP_{PTT,Cal} - BP_{Cal} \tag{10.3}$$

This coefficient is used to correct the calculated value in this one point calibrated system and provide an absolute value for the systolic blood pressure of the user. Patzak *et al.* [26] developed continuous blood pressure measurement using PTT and considered a comparative argument to intra-arterial measurement in real-time for more stability and higher accuracy. The research study [26] related the user's pulse wave velocity to their blood pressure using PWV and systolic blood pressure data obtained from 13 subjects. This function consists of an exponential term, a second non-linear term, and finally the correction constant calculated during the calibration procedure. This function is shown in (10.4).

$$\text{BP} = 700\ \text{PWV} + 766,000\ \text{PWV}^9 - \text{CC}\ [\text{mmHg}] \tag{10.4}$$

10.3.4 Vital sign monitoring system design and modelling

The QRS complex was important in the development of the continuous blood pressure measurement application, especially the amplitude peak of the R wave. Another key parameter was Photoplethysmogram (PPG), which is typically an optically obtained plethysmogram. The plethysmogram measurement is the capacity change of volume within an organ in the body, or the whole body itself. PPG acts as the measurement of the change in cardiac volume, in this case. This operation is implemented by using a pulse oximeter much like the ones used for blood oxygen saturation however the main difference is the pulse detection by transmission or reflection of light through the skin in the photodiode.

10.3.5 Falls risk assessment

Integration of changes in blood pressure and other vital signs into the falls risk assessment system gives an enormous advantage to the proposed multifactorial falls risk assessment model in identification and classification of falls risk. Integration of vital signs has been poorly addressed in the literature [27,28]. However, there is evidence for concrete association between the vital sign(s) and falls [29]. One of the expert rules or conditions adopted in the proposed fuzzy-logic based model was the drop of systolic blood pressure for the case of postural hypotension such that:

> A fall of more than 20 mmHg in systolic blood pressure and/or more than 10 mmHg in diastolic blood pressure when standing (compared to the sitting blood pressure) indicates risk of fall [29].

A direct link between the changes in blood pressure and falls assessment model was implemented that contribute to the falls risk assessment. Direct and indirect links between the ECG and PPG have been maintained throughout the design and development phases due to the fact that the clinical situation, particularly of hospitalised patients, is often variable (unstable) over days or even hours. The integration of the proposed model with real-time vital signs towards the falls risk assessment has given the proposed model a unique tool in falls risk assessment.

The pattern recognition classifier accurately detects and classifies the difference between falls, a stumble to the right and left, sitting on the chair and a fall onto a chair. A falls detection model using motion data alone as well as a combination of motion data and vital signs was also explored [30].

Considering users' need and clinicians' preferences, it was found that non-invasive, wireless and body-worn sensors do provide a better solution in the design of such falls risk assessment model. In the hospital or residential aged care facility, there would be a need for an alarm-type system that sends a nurse urgent messages to check patient's immediate status – hopefully this can then prevent a fall that may be due to "feeling faint" or drop of blood pressure. In the community as operating on a slower alarm system – alerting on-duty physicians that this person is deteriorating in terms of vital signs/mobility and needs to be semi-urgently reassessed.

10.4 Application development and system performance

The *pulse transit time* is defined as the time delay between the R-wave of the ECG and the arrival of a pulse wave from the pulse oximeter in the same cardiac cycle. This satisfies the need for the measurement to come from two separate arterial sites while also being in the same cardiac cycle. PPT then incorporates both the devices (ECG activity monitor and Pulse oximeter). PTT has been shown to be quasi-linear to low BP values, but increase exponentially at higher pressures. It is now proven that several factors such as age, gender, and cardiovascular risk factors greatly influence the PWV values and can therefore only be used for measuring relative changes in BP. Conversely, if the individual PWV–BP relation and calibration can be completed, the system would allow for the absolute BP to be measured using the PTT. This method can be very time-consuming and arduous therefore a one-point calibration of the PWV–BP relation was implemented, for faster processing and higher accuracy. Figure 10.2 shows the ECG and pulse wave with ECG peaks and pulse oximeter peaks detection for faster processing on incoming device data.

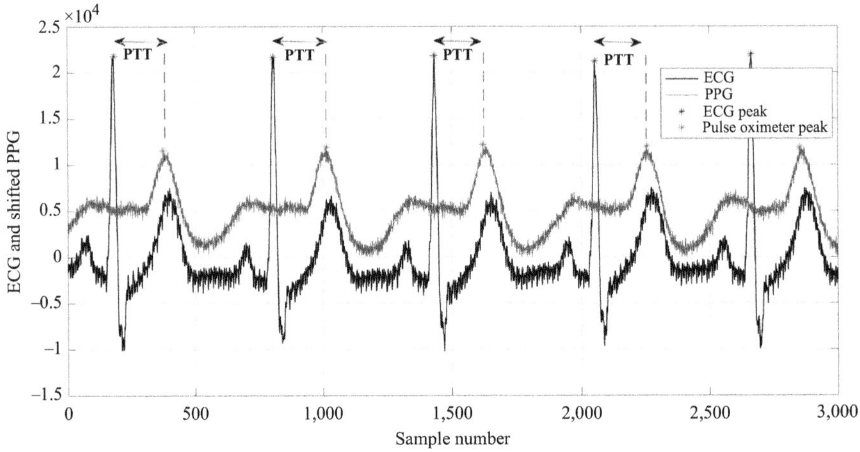

Figure 10.2 ECG and pulse oximeter peaks detection for faster and accurate calculations

10.4.1 ECG and PPG data handling

The incoming data packets of ECG and PPG are extracted and displayed on the monitoring screen, the user is allowed to save the data for feature extraction as well as data analysis. The monitoring application also allows for reviewing data, time-based trends, and displaying the history activity of the application. The height is used in the application for the use of measuring continuous BP. An object query into the current user was implemented returning the height in a string format; this allows each user to use their personal measurements such as height in this instance.

10.4.2 Cloud-based data storage and data security

High importance is given to the information exchange and this research aims to bring "the right information at the right time to the right place". This requires a central storage database that is easily accessible to various mobile and medical monitoring devices. Database access is handled by the application "backend". Third party backends provide professional data management with world class security and reliability. There were several options available in the commercial as well as research space, however after closer inspection of available backend systems, "Parse" was selected as the most suitable backend system to the standard and open information aim of this research project due to the high level of support and low learning curve.

The data storage protocols were used throughout the application form the login activities all the way through to saving the PPG and ECG data during the monitoring activity. A secure and safe web-based account is the only access to the web console or web application where all vital and user sensitive information can be viewed. Once the web application was created, a unique application ID is created for each user and that unique ID is linked to the Parse web application and the mobile monitoring application. This is initialised in an activity which extends the application (as Parse is the extension). The extension allows the initialisation to occur whenever the application is started, with or without wireless network availability. Both applications (web and mobile) are ready to start saving the incoming raw data as well as processed continuous blood pressure data. As the Parse SDK is object orientated, the coding is very much similar to that used for the android SDK.

10.4.3 User-centric approach

The Android application is developed with high user-centric approach and user engagement so that the monitoring application is best tailored for secondary care users. It is clear from the literature review [31] that most of the smartphone application do not meet the user centric acceptance criteria and standards, thus majority of the smartphone-based healthcare applications received poor user-centric rating. Based on this challenge, we emphasised user acceptability into our development process, leveraging learnings from the literature as well as commercially successful applications available in the market [31–33].

One of the common requirements is that, the application context should be easily understood by the users [34]. Since the application was being targeted at a secondary care, it was designed to be as simple to use as possible and at the same time as informative as possible. The application has an intuitive user experience with wizards implemented with clear instructions. This improves the user experience greatly since there is no need to look at other sources to figure out how the application and devices function. Finally, the responsiveness of the application is fast and of the greatest standard with good connectivity to the assigned devices. The navigation between screens is really smooth and there is no delay within the application functionality. Figure 10.3 shows the proposed application screen with systolic blood pressure, heart beats per minute, and blood oxygen readings in real-time from various connected medical devices. Colour coded images, icons, and graphical views are used for enhanced user experience and maintain compatibility with the current mode of paper-based data collection process.

10.5 Discussion and conclusion

The developed smartphone application evolved during implementation of different phases of this research, emphasising that each iteration provided significant improvement in development of the application. Despite the proliferation and almost ubiquitous use of mobile devices, the usability of mobile websites and applications can almost match the usability of desktop websites. Our approach to the mobile app usability testing can be helpful in addressing some of the barriers to assessing the usability of mobile devices which have been previously noted such as lack of big size memory, small screen space, and poor graphical displays [35].

Time delay and data synchronisations were critical challenges to overcome in order to use the real-time PPT and ECG data for further processing. This research

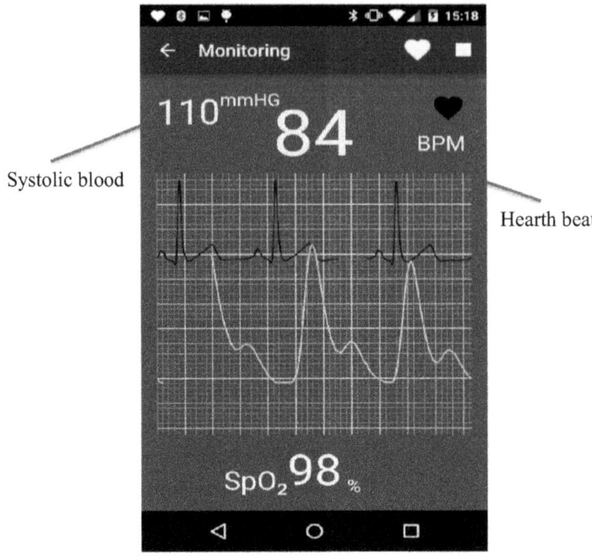

Figure 10.3 Real-time monitoring of blood pressure, heartbeat and oxygen saturation levels with graphical view and decision support

adopted Bluetooth/IEEE 802.15.4 wireless technologies for real-time sensing and time synchronisation. The proposed monitoring application adopted and used open and standard platforms for mobile applications and medical monitoring devices for connectivity to different types of devices and platforms using IEEE standards for wireless connectivity. This adoption would expand the range of health extremities that can be monitored, as well as allowing more new concepts to be tried and tested using this type of software interface. Along with support for more devices, a multi-brand diversity across medical equipment would provide a greater range and a more universal type of mobile application going forward.

The application was successful in its key goal of connecting different medical monitoring devices, receiving information, recording, processing, and displaying of data. The attempted method of synchronisation, using the number of samples received and setting the ECG transmission time as a base line, can overcome this challenge but it also leads to the PTT times not being constant after the connections are restarted. Thus, more accurate and consistent real-time detection of instantaneous PTT is required. The critical element is the adoption and use of standard and best practice approach/methods and synchronisation between the devices. Moreover, such healthcare apps could pose some safety risks to the public and patients if they result in clinical decision-making.

Apart from the above challenges, further research enhancements could be conducted on the following technological gaps in the current mobile healthcare applications domain. Firstly, clinicians and patients are the underused resources in mobile applications design and development; early collaboration of developers and clinicians along with the target users are critical towards the successful healthcare applications being implemented in the hospital care settings. Secondly, appropriate use or representation of information including data analysis, interpretation, translation, integration, and processing should be accurate and presented to the medical professional in a simple and easy format. Due to the streaming disparate coming originating from multiple medical monitoring devices, it is now a critical task to represent the raw data as meaningful or useful to the clinician.

Nonetheless, there are numerous benefits of successfully implementing continuous non-invasive blood pressure monitoring on a mobile device. Such an application would allow short-term blood pressure changes to be monitored and could help in the falls prevention and early patient deterioration.

References

[1] Brown, I. and Adams, A.A., 'The ethical challenges of ubiquitous healthcare', *International Review of Information Ethics*, 2007, 8(12), pp. 53–60.

[2] Baig, M.M., Gholamhosseini, H., and Connolly, M.J., 'Mobile healthcare applications: system design review, critical issues and challenges', *Australasian Physical & Engineering Sciences in Medicine*, 2015, 38(1), pp. 23–38.

[3] Baig, M.M. and Gholamhosseini, H., 'Smart health monitoring systems: an overview of design and modeling', *Journal of Medical Systems*, 2013, 37(2), p. 98.

[4] Silva, B.M., Rodrigues, J.J., de la Torre Díez, I., López-Coronado, M., and Saleem, K., 'Mobile-health: a review of current state in 2015', *Journal of Biomedical Informatics*, 2015, 56, pp. 265–272.

[5] Ozkaynak, M. and Brennan, P., 'An observation tool for studying patient-oriented workflow in hospital emergency departments', *Methods of Information in Medicine*, 2013, 52(6), pp. 503–513.

[6] Holzinger, A., Kosec, P., Schwantzer, G., Debevc, M., Hofmann-Wellenhof, R., and Frühauf, J., 'Design and development of a mobile computer application to reengineer workflows in the hospital and the methodology to evaluate its effectiveness', *Journal of Biomedical Informatics*, 2011, 44(6), pp. 968–977.

[7] Lee, B.M., 'Registration protocol for health Iot platform to share the use of medical devices', *International Journal of Bio-Science and Bio-Technology*, 2015, 7(4), pp. 1–10.

[8] Mukhopadhyay, S.C., 'Wearable sensors for human activity monitoring: a review', *IEEE Sensors Journal*, 2015, 15(3), pp. 1321–1330.

[9] Goldberg, E.M. and Levy, P.D., 'New approaches to evaluating and monitoring blood pressure', *Current Hypertension Reports*, 2016, 18(6), pp. 1–7.

[10] Buxi, D., Redouté, J.-M., and Yuce, M.R., 'A survey on signals and systems in ambulatory blood pressure monitoring using pulse transit time', *Physiological Measurement*, 2015, 36(3), pp. R1–R26.

[11] Baig, M.M., Gholamhosseini, H., and Connolly, M.J., 'A comprehensive survey of wearable and wireless ECG monitoring systems for older adults', *Medical & Biological Engineering & Computing*, 2013, 51(5), pp. 485–495.
[12] McColl, L.D., Rideout, P.E., Parmar, T.N., and Abba-Aji, A., 'Peer support intervention through mobile application: an integrative literature review and future directions', *Canadian Psychology/Psychologie Canadienne*, 2014, 55(4), pp. 250–257.
[13] Maass, W. and Varshney, U., 'Design and evaluation of ubiquitous information systems and use in healthcare', *Decision Support Systems*, 2012, 54(1), pp. 597–609.
[14] Volk, R.J., Llewellyn-Thomas, H., Stacey, D., and Elwyn, G., 'Ten years of the international patient decision aid standards collaboration: evolution of the core dimensions for assessing the quality of patient decision aids', *BMC Medical Informatics and Decision Making*, 2013, 13(2), p. S1.
[15] Malvey, D. and Slovensky, D.J., 'mHealth products, markets, and trends', mHealth*: Transforming Healthcare* (Springer, New York, 2014).
[16] Friesen, M.R., Hamel, C., and McLeod, R.D., 'A mHealth application for chronic wound care: findings of a user trial', *International Journal of Environmental Research and Public Health*, 2013, 10(11), pp. 6199–6214.
[17] Black, J., Baharestani, M.M., Cuddigan, J., *et al.*, 'National pressure ulcer advisory panel's updated pressure ulcer staging system', *Advances in Skin & Wound Care*, 2007, 20(5), pp. 269–274.
[18] Bergstrom, N., Braden, B.J., Laguzza, A., and Holman, V., 'The Braden scale for predicting pressure sore risk', *Nursing Research*, 1987, 36(4), pp. 205–210.
[19] Harris, C., Bates-Jensen, B., Parslow, N., Raizman, R., Singh, M., and Ketchen, R., 'Bates-Jensen wound assessment tool: pictorial guide validation project', *Journal of Wound Ostomy & Continence Nursing*, 2010, 37(3), pp. 253–259.
[20] Luxton, D.D., Kayl, R.A., and Mishkind, M.C., 'mHealth data security: the need for HIPAA-compliant standardization', *Telemedicine and e-Health*, 2012, 18(4), pp. 284–288.
[21] Bickmore, T.W., Silliman, R.A., Nelson, K., *et al.*, 'A randomized controlled trial of an automated exercise coach for older adults', *Journal of the American Geriatrics Society*, 2013, 61(10), pp. 1676–1683.
[22] Fromme, E.K., Kenworthy-Heinige, T., and Hribar, M., 'Developing an easy-to-use tablet computer application for assessing patient-reported outcomes in patients with cancer', *Supportive Care in Cancer*, 2011, 19(6), pp. 815–822.
[23] Steinhubl, S.R., Muse, E.D., and Topol, E.J., 'Can mobile health technologies transform health care?', *JAMA*, 2013, 310(22), pp. 2395–2396.
[24] Petersen, C., Adams, S.A., and DeMuro, P.R., 'mHealth: don't forget all the stakeholders in the business case', *Medicine 2.0*, 2015, 4(2), p. e4.
[25] Nonin Medical, Inc. "Onyx II, Model 9560-fingertip pulse oximeter." (2016). Accessed 28 April 28 2017. http://www.nonin.com/PulseOximetry/Fingertip/Onyx9560.

[26] Patzak, A., Mendoza, Y., Gesche, H., and Konermann, M., 'Continuous blood pressure measurement using the pulse transit time: comparison to intra-arterial measurement', *Blood Pressure*, 2015, 24(4), pp. 217–221.

[27] Vassallo, M., Mallela, S.K., Williams, A., Kwan, J., Allen, S., and Sharma, J.C., 'Fall risk factors in elderly patients with cognitive impairment on rehabilitation wards', *Geriatrics & Gerontology International*, 2009, 9(1), pp. 41–46.

[28] Oliver, D., 'Falls risk-prediction tools for hospital inpatients. Time to put them to bed?', *Age and Ageing*, 2008, 37(3), pp. 248–250.

[29] Naschitz, J.E. and Rosner, I., 'Orthostatic hypotension: framework of the syndrome', *Postgraduate Medical Journal*, 2007, 83(983), pp. 568–574.

[30] Baig, M.M., Gholamhosseini, H., and Connolly, M.J., 'Falls risk assessment for hospitalised older adults: a combination of motion data and vital signs', *Aging Clinical and Experimental Research*, 2016, 28(6), pp. 1159–1168.

[31] Fruhling, A.L., Raman, S., and McGrath, S., 'Mobile healthcare user interface design application strategies', in Eren, H. and Webster, J. (eds.), *Telehealth and Mobile Health* (CRC Press, Boca Raton, FL, 2015)

[32] Mosa, A.S.M., Yoo, I., and Sheets, L., 'A systematic review of healthcare applications for smartphones', *BMC Medical Informatics and Decision Making*, 2012, 12(1), p. 67.

[33] Dinh, H.T., Lee, C., Niyato, D., and Wang, P., 'A survey of mobile cloud computing: architecture, applications, and approaches', *Wireless Communications and Mobile Computing*, 2013, 13(18), pp. 1587–1611.

[34] Peischl, B., Ferk, M., and Holzinger, A., 'The fine art of user-centered software development', *Software Quality Journal*, 2015, 23(3), pp. 509–536.

[35] Sheehan, B., Lee, Y., Rodriguez, M., Tiase, V., and Schnall, R., 'A comparison of usability factors of four mobile devices for accessing healthcare information by adolescents', *Applied Clinical Informatics*, 2012, 3(4), pp. 356–366.

Index

www.ingramcontent.com/pod-product-compliance
Ingram Content Group UK Ltd.
Pitfield, Milton Keynes, MK11 3LW, UK
UKHW020809290926
15470UKWH00003B/1045

9 781785 611506